THE NEUROLEPTIC MALIGNANT SYNDROME AND RELATED CONDITIONS

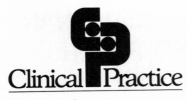

Clinical Practice

Number 6

Judith H. Gold, M.D., F.R.C.P.(C)
Series Editor

THE NEUROLEPTIC MALIGNANT SYNDROME AND RELATED CONDITIONS

ARTHUR LAZARUS, M.D.

Clinical Assistant Professor of Psychiatry, Temple University
School of Medicine; and Philadelphia Psychiatric Center

STEPHAN C. MANN, M.D.

Clinical Assistant Professor of Psychiatry, University of
Pennsylvania; and V.A. Medical Center, Philadelphia

STANLEY N. CAROFF, M.D.

Associate Professor of Psychiatry, University of Pennsylvania;
and V.A. Medical Center, Philadelphia

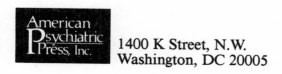 1400 K Street, N.W.
Washington, DC 20005

Note: The authors have worked to ensure that all information in this book concerning drug dosages, schedules, and routes of administration is accurate as of the time of publication and consistent with standards set by the U.S. Food and Drug Administration and the general medical community. As medical research and practice advance, however, therapeutic standards may change. For this reason and because human and mechanical errors sometimes occur, we recommend that readers follow the advice of a physician who is directly involved in their care or the care of a member of the family.

Books published by the American Psychiatric Press, Inc., represent the views and opinions of the individual authors and do not necessarily represent the policies and opinions of the Press or the American Psychiatric Association.

Library of Congress Cataloging-in-Publication Data

Lazarus, Arthur, 1954-
    The neuroleptic malignant syndrome and related conditions / Arthur Lazarus, Stephan C. Mann, Stanley N. Caroff.
        p.   cm.—(The Clinical practice series ; no. 6)
    Bibliography: p.
    ISBN 0-88048-134-X (alk. paper).
    1. Psychotropic drugs—Side effects.   I. Mann, Stephan C., 1948-   . II. Caroff, Stanley N., 1949- . III. Title. IV. Series:
Clinical practice series (Washington, D.C.) ; no. 6.
    [DNLM: 1. Catatonia.   2. Malignant Hyperthermia.
3. Neuroleptic Malignant Syndrome.   4. Tranquilizing Agents, Major—adverse effects.   WL 307 L431n]
RM315.L35 1988
615'.788—dc19
DNLM/DLC   88-24242
for Library of Congress   CIP

Contents

Introduction
to the Clinical Practice Series

*O*ver the years of its existence the series of monographs entitled *Clinical Insights* gradually became focused on providing current, factual, and theoretical material of interest to the clinician working outside of a hospital setting. To reflect this orientation, the name of the Series has been changed to *Clinical Practice.*

The Clinical Practice Series will provide readers with books that give the mental health clinician a practical clinical approach to a variety of psychiatric problems. These books will provide up-to-date literature reviews and emphasize the most recent treatment methods. Thus, the publications in the Series will interest clinicians working both in psychiatry and in the other mental health professions.

Each year a number of books will be published dealing with all aspects of clinical practice. In addition, from time to time when appropriate, the publications may be revised and updated. Thus, the Series will provide quick access to relevant and important areas of psychiatric practice. Some books in the Series will be authored by a person considered to be an expert in that particular area; others will be edited by such an expert who will also draw together other knowledgeable authors to produce a comprehensive overview of that topic.

Some of the books in the Clinical Practice Series will have their foundation in presentations at an Annual Meeting of the American Psychiatric Association. All will contain the most recently available information on the subjects discussed. Theoretical and scientific data will be applied to clinical situations, and case illustrations will be utilized in order to make the material even more relevant for the practitioner. Thus, the Clinical Practice Series should provide educational reading in a compact format especially written for the mental health clinician–psychiatrist.

All clinicians working with patients requiring the use of neuroleptics are troubled by the occurrence of side effects. One of the most difficult and troubling of these is the Neuroleptic Malignant Syndrome. The authors of this monograph present a thorough review of all the present research in the field and offer advice to the clinician in dealing with this difficult clinical situation. This monograph is a valuable addition to our Clinical Practice Series in its up-to-date clinical approach to this condition.

Judith H. Gold, M.D., F.R.C.P.(C)
Series Editor,
Clinical Practice Series

Preface

*T*he introduction of psychotropic medication, and neuroleptics in particular, has been viewed as one of the great advances in modern psychiatry. Neuroleptic drugs have played a major role in the treatment of schizophrenia and other psychotic disorders, allowing large numbers of patients to receive community-based and other ambulatory treatments. Although neuroleptics do not cure schizophrenia, they have decreased disability and suffering associated with the illness, and have made it possible for many patients to enjoy more independent and productive lives.

Shortly after neuroleptics were in clinical use, however, it became apparent that these drugs had many undesirable side effects, some inseparable from their therapeutic effects. One such example is tardive dyskinesia, an involuntary movement disorder associated with long-term neuroleptic therapy. Although the clinical manifestations of tardive dyskinesia were first described in the late 1950s, it was not until recently that this condition was given more serious consideration. Increasing concerns over the risk of tardive dyskinesia have led to a reevaluation of dosage and treatment strategies in the maintenance treatment of psychotic disorders, and have underscored the need to develop antipsychotic drugs with fewer untoward effects.

Now, in addition to tardive dyskinesia, other neuroleptic-induced disorders have become a pressing concern. Of particular note are acute, idiosyncratic extrapyramidal reactions and neuroleptic-related disturbances in thermoregulation and autonomic function. The neuroleptic malignant syndrome (NMS) is a condition characterized by such impairments. It is clear that neuroleptic drugs may cause a "malignant syndrome" and that this syndrome presents a serious obstacle to the treatment of some patients who require neuroleptic therapy. In fact, NMS may be as troublesome, and certainly more acutely dangerous, a complication of antipsychotic drug therapy as is tardive dyskinesia. In some individuals at risk for recurrent episodes of NMS, clinicians may be faced with the same dilemma they find themselves in when treating a patient with tardive dyskinesia: withholding neuroleptics at the expense of chronic psychosis, providing alternative treatment that is often less than satisfactory, or risking recurrence of NMS associated with the readministration of neuroleptic drugs.

We decided to write this book for several reasons. First and foremost is the fact that NMS is rare, has been slow to receive proper recognition, and continues to generate controversy. The topic has been largely neglected in contemporary psychiatric texts. Most clinicians we have encountered are unaware of the syndrome or are only vaguely cognizant of it. Some have acknowledged dealing with patients with NMS in retrospect, once they have become familiar with the syndrome. On the other hand, some investigators familiar with NMS and similar conditions have begun to develop diverse strategies for understanding and treating this disorder.

We expect that an increased appreciation of NMS and related syndromes will lead to improved diagnostic acuity, more effective therapy, and better preventive measures. A reduction in morbidity resulting from adverse reactions to neuroleptic drugs may increase acceptance of neuroleptics among patients and society, and lessen any threat these reactions may pose to the vitality of neuroleptic prescribing. Greater clinical understanding of adverse reactions caused by neuroleptics may help stem the tide of increasing malpractice litigation in this area.

Because many features of NMS overlap with several other conditions directly or indirectly related to neuroleptic therapy, the potential for confusion is significant. Although there is no deficit of articles on NMS and other similar conditions, the interested clinician must cull the American and foreign literature and at best can obtain information in piecemeal fashion based largely on limited anecdotal experiences. We anticipate that this book will be a useful resource and serve as a timely, balanced, and comprehensive synthesis of available data. The material may also provide a valuable framework for guiding future research and developing more innovative treatments.

Finally, we hope that a broad and scientific review of these rare toxic reactions may provide fresh insight into the clinical pharmacology and mechanisms of action of neuroleptic drugs.

From both a clinical and research point of view, this book should have multidisciplinary appeal because neuroleptic drugs are in widespread use. Our intended audience is not only psychiatrists and mental health professionals, but also neurologists, internists, anesthesiologists, neurophysiologists, and pharmacologists. We have seen various neuroscientists in attendance at symposia and paper sessions on NMS at recent meetings of the American Psychiatric Association. All have shared with us their enthusiasm, expertise, and quest for further knowledge. We hope this monograph captures the spirit embodied in those meetings, not only for our colleagues but for all readers.

Our sincere thanks go to Rita Stewart, Phyllis Smith, and Joanne Loguidici for their skillful secretarial assistance and manuscript preparation.

This book is lovingly dedicated to our wives, Cheryl, Maureen, and Rosalind, and to our children.

Chapter 1
The Neuroleptic Malignant Syndrome

Chapter 1

The Neuroleptic Malignant Syndrome

*T*he safety and efficacy of neuroleptics in the management of psychotic patients has been well established through more than 30 years of experience with these drugs. Side effects produced by neuroleptics are relatively predictable, and although unpleasant for the patient, are rarely life-threatening. One notable exception is the neuroleptic malignant syndrome (NMS), an often misdiagnosed and sometimes fatal complication of antipsychotic drug therapy. Despite having gained considerable awareness among some physicians, NMS still thwarts therapeutic efforts of many who are unfamiliar with the syndrome.

Although NMS or its equivalent under other synonyms has been diagnosed for more than 25 years, it remains an elusive entity, difficult to define, and in some cases inappropriately labeled. There is considerable controversy over its key features, and some investigators (Cohen et al. 1987; Levinson and Simpson 1986) have even questioned its diagnostic validity. Moreover, although many explanations of its pathogenesis have been advanced, none of them appears to explain all aspects of the syndrome. The occurrence of NMS continues to raise many questions regarding its etiology and relationship to lethal catatonia, heatstroke, malignant hyperthermia, and hyperthermic syndromes associated with other pharmacologic agents.

However, substantial clinical data have accumulated based on numerous case reports and several reviews of the subject. In addition, some investigators have formulated hypotheses about NMS and have begun to test these

3

experimentally. Given these considerations, it becomes important for physicians to be familiar with NMS and current concepts regarding its diagnosis, pathogenesis, and treatment.

Historical Background

The term *syndrome malin* had long been used in France as a nonspecific medical term referring to a fulminant, neurovegetative state with impending disaster. As a purely descriptive term, *syndrome malin* had many etiologies. It was often associated with fever and fatal infectious processes (Fourrier 1965). Delay and associates (1962) employed the term *syndrome malin des neuroleptiques* when similar alarming findings were observed in neuroleptic-treated patients: pallor, hyperthermia, and respiratory and psychomotor abnormalities.

The English translation of *syndrome malin des neuroleptiques*—"neuroleptic malignant syndrome"—first appeared in 1968. Delay and Deniker (1968) considered NMS "the most serious but also the rarest and least known of the complications of neuroleptic chemotherapy" (p. 258). It should be noted that what has been lost in translation and often misunderstood is the fact that the syndrome, not the neuroleptic, is "malignant."

Prior to the 1960s, clinical descriptions of cases resembling NMS reported in American literature were not formally diagnosed as NMS. In 1956 Cohen described his experience with 1,400 patients treated with chlorpromazine (40 to 2500 mg/day) over a 14-month period. Complications included fever in the absence of infection, parkinsonism, renal insufficiency, facial pallor, pulmonary hypostasis, and other signs often seen in NMS. Kinross-Wright (1958) reported NMS-like episodes in two young adults treated with trifluoperazine, attributed these reactions to massive inhibition of brain-stem function, and concluded that early recognition and immediate drug withdrawal were mandatory for a favorable outcome. Preston (1959) described six patients

4

treated with therapeutic doses of phenothiazines who developed prominent neuromuscular abnormalities of the head and neck, autonomic impairment, and confusion. Fever was present in two patients, one of whom died; an autopsy revealed no apparent cause of death. May (1959) reported phenothiazine-induced catatonic-like states in two patients that were associated with autonomic disturbances, particularly sialorrhea and respiratory changes, but without fever. In all of these cases the adverse effects of neuroleptics were thought to be secondary to their actions in the central nervous system (CNS). It was believed that affected individuals were predisposed on an allergic basis or, in some cases, on the basis of their young age. The toxic reaction developed by these patients was not dose dependent.

Interest and increased awareness in febrile catatonic states associated with neuroleptic administration was quite evident by the mid-1970s. At this time, NMS had been fairly well reported in France, Japan, and England. Several American authors, cognizant of the French reports, also began to use the term *neuroleptic malignant syndrome* to describe similar cases in the United States.

Meltzer (1973) described a 21-year-old psychotic college student who became mute, immobile, and incontinent 24 hours after she was given a subcutaneous injection of fluphenazine enanthate (25 mg). She then developed severe muscular rigidity, hyperpyrexia (103° F), and increased levels of serum creatine phosphokinase (CPK). She became comatose. The syndrome resolved mainly with supportive treatment. Rechallenge with fluphenazine enanthate and other neuroleptics did not cause recurrence of symptoms.

Both Meltzer (1973), and Weinberger and Kelly (1977) in a similar case, called attention to the clinical aspects of NMS and noted the difficulty in distinguishing it from Stauder's (1934) "lethal catatonia," an identical condition described early in the century and apparently unrelated to neuroleptic therapy (see Chapter 5). Powers and associates (1976) reported a case of chlorpromazine-induced NMS, also clinically indistinguishable from lethal catatonia, successfully treated with electroconvulsive therapy (ECT) "despite the usual practice of not administering ECT in the presence of fever" (p. 360).

Caroff (1980) published a frequently cited review of NMS in English in 1980. He examined more than 60 cases described in the world literature at that time, and suggested that NMS was seriously underrecognized and underdiagnosed. Using diagnostic criteria similar to those proposed by Delay and Deniker (1968) (i.e., hyperthermia, rigidity, altered consciousness, and autonomic instability), he cited reports that suggested NMS may occur as frequently as 0.5 to 1 percent of neuroleptic-treated patients and may culminate in death in 20 percent of cases. In his survey of clinical material available at the time, Caroff (1980) also outlined demographic characteristics of affected patients and the major clinical features and course of NMS.

Consistent with earlier reports, Caroff (1980) suggested that NMS could be distinguished from neuroleptic-related heatstroke, appeared to be similar to malignant hyperthermia, and resembled lethal catatonia, which he suggested was a nonspecific, descriptive syndrome. The association between these conditions and hyperthermic syndromes related to other drugs led Caroff (1980) to propose that NMS may be the neuroleptic-induced subtype of a more generalized spectrum of hyperthermic disorders that could be induced in susceptible patients by a variety of pharmacologic agents.

By 1986, more than 300 cases of NMS had been reported in the literature (Pearlman 1986). Also in 1986, the term *neuroleptic malignant syndrome* was included as a specific medical heading in *Index Medicus*. It had previously been cross-indexed under headings such as "basal ganglia diseases," "fever," "muscle rigidity," and "tranquilizing agents." The *Physician's Desk Reference* did not report NMS as an adverse reaction of neuroleptic therapy until 1985.

It is not clear why, until recently, NMS remained esoteric, or why it received belated recognition in the United

States. In this regard, one sees a parallel between NMS and tardive dyskinesia. Yet tardive dyskinesia generally takes years to develop, whereas NMS has a dramatic presentation and usually occurs during the early phase of treatment. It is disconcerting that despite the widespread use of neuroleptics, these two relatively severe reactions were not recognized earlier. Possible reasons for the belated recognition of NMS may involve the preponderance of early reports and reviews in non-English languages and the failure to distinguish signs and symptoms of NMS from underlying psychogenic conditions, benign extrapyramidal reactions, and medical complications or medical illnesses that resemble NMS.

Incidence

Although the syndrome was originally thought to be rare, case reports of NMS have increased substantially over the last several years. In New York, Greenberg and Gujavarty (1985) observed three cases in 4 months in a 30-bed university admission service. Janati and Webb (1986) reported four patients with NMS who were admitted to the medical intensive care unit at the Little Rock Veterans Administration Medical Center between January and April of 1984. Kimsey et al. (1983) identified six instances of NMS in five patients in 1 year at Rusk State Hospital, Texas. Nine cases of NMS were observed in 2 years at the Medical College of Wisconsin hospitals (Harsch 1987). In France, Fabre and colleagues (1977) noted seven cases in a single year, and Destée and associates (1980) reported 31 cases over a 9-year period. In the single largest series to date, which includes specific clinical data, Itoh et al. (1977) in Japan described 14 cases of NMS observed over a 5-year period. However, none of these studies provided an incidence rate; the total number of patients at risk during these time periods was not determined.

Other reports have provided data that allow an estimation of the incidence in NMS (Table 1.1). The incidence of

NMS in these studies varied from 0.02 to 3.23 percent, suggesting that NMS may occur on average at a rate as high as 1 percent, as originally estimated (Caroff 1980; Delay et al. 1962). Variations in incidence, which ranged over a hundredfold between investigators, may be due to several factors, including the level of awareness and experience of clinicians, differences in populations and clinical settings, and use of different diagnostic criteria. For example, fever and muscle rigidity initially may not be recognized as associated with neuroleptic use. Even more likely, early warning signs of NMS, such as autonomic instability, may not be recognized and may resolve before the diagnosis is considered (Addonizio et al. 1986). Conversely, in view of the lack of consensus on diagnostic criteria, diagnosis of false positive cases with few or minor symptoms of NMS may inflate estimates of the incidence of the disorder. Because the number of patients in some of the studies is relatively small, diagnostic changes in only a few cases could significantly alter the incidence. Also, the existence of significant cultural effects on the dosage tolerance and potential for neuroleptic toxicity (Lin et al. 1986) may influence the incidence of NMS. Thus more precise estimates of the incidence of NMS depend on the development of standardized, reliable diagnostic criteria

TABLE 1.1. Incidence of NMS

Reference	N	NMS	%
Delay et al. (1960)	62	2	3.23
Singh (1981)	1,500	3	0.20
Neppe (1984)	6,000	1	0.02
Sukanova (1985)	4,000	6	0.15
Shalev and Munitz (1986)	1,250	5	0.40
Boyer (1986)	?	?	0.40
Addonizio et al. (1986)	82	2	2.44
Pope et al. (1986b)	483	7	1.45
Keck et al. (1987)	679	6	0.88
Gelenberg et al. (1988)	1,470	1	0.07

Note. Mean ± SD = 0.9 ± 1.1.

and large-scale, prospective studies to monitor patients
undergoing neuroleptic treatment.

Onset and Predisposing Factors

Neuroleptic Drugs

Neuroleptics from all classes of antipsychotic drugs have been
associated with NMS. In approximately one-third of cases,
patients have received two or more neuroleptic drugs
(Addonizio et al. 1987; Kurlan et al. 1984), making it difficult
to distinguish the effects of individual drugs.

The majority of cases of NMS occur in patients treated
with high-potency neuroleptics, particularly haloperidol,
which has been associated with nearly half of all reported
cases (Table 1.2). This observation has led many authors to
conclude that patients receiving high-potency neuroleptics
are at increased risk of developing NMS. Alternative
explanations may be possible, however, because high-potency
neuroleptics may be prescribed more frequently and at higher

TABLE 1.2. Neuroleptics Taken Within One Week of NMS Episodes

Drug	Drug Episodes	Single Drug	Daily Dose (mg)[a]
Haloperidol	102	61	31 ± 32
Chlorpromazine	34	10	694 ± 88
Fluphenazine (depot)	23	14	44 ± 29[b]
Trifluoperazine	15	9	30 ± 28
Fluphenazine	14	8	14 ± 14
Thioridazine	14	4	271 ± 227
Thiothixene	13	8	31 ± 15
Other neuroleptics[c]	68	24	————

Note. Based on case reports of 219 patients reported between 1980–1987
in which these drug data could be ascertained.
[a] Mean ± SD, single drug episodes only.
[b] Weekly.
[c] Includes drugs not currently available in the United States.

milligram equivalent dosages than low-potency neuroleptics (Baldessarini et al. 1984). Also, high-potency antipsychotics may be more likely to be given to medically ill or young acutely psychotic patients who may be at higher risk of developing NMS (Caroff 1980; Levenson 1985). However, NMS may be caused by low-potency drugs and even atypical agents such as reserpine (Haggerty et al. 1987) and clozapine (Pope et al. 1986a).

Shalev and Munitz (1986) suggested that the onset of NMS was associated with a high rate of neuroleptic loading, equivalent to increasing daily therapy by approximately 500 to 700 mg of chlorpromazine. In addition, perhaps related to the rate of loading (Shalev and Munitz 1986), the intramuscular and intravenous routes of administration seem to potentiate the development of NMS (Itoh et al. 1977; Lew and Tollefson 1983). Kirkpatrick and Edelsohn (1985) found that NMS was correlated with high doses of neuroleptics, rather than rate of increase, although the validity of their results was questioned by Pearlman (1986). Overall, NMS has been reported with a wide range of doses and does not appear to be dose related; it usually occurs at therapeutic rather than toxic doses (cf. Table 1.2). Neuroleptic blood levels, when measured, have been within reported normal limits (Greenberg and Gorelick 1986; Lazarus 1986c; Granato et al. 1983; Hashimoto et al. 1984).

Some investigators (Allan and White 1972; Caroff 1980; Grunhaus et al. 1979) have pointed out potential dangers for patients who develop NMS while receiving depot neuroleptics. All six cases of NMS reported by Kimsey et al. (1983) involved the administration of fluphenazine decanoate. Caroff's (1980) review indicated that long-acting fluphenazine compounds were associated with increased mortality in NMS, perhaps because the long half-life of these agents results in greater duration of exposure to the risk of medical complications. Pearlman (1986) confirmed the longer duration and morbidity of NMS with depot neuroleptics but not an increased mortality. Although at this time evidence is not conclusive for increased incidence or mortality from NMS in relation to treatment with depot drugs, it would seem prudent to monitor the use of long-acting neuroleptics carefully in view of the longer duration and morbidity of NMS secondary to these drugs.

More than half of cases of NMS involve the concomitant administration of medication other than neuroleptics (e.g., lithium carbonate, tricyclic antidepressants, antiparkinsonian medications, and benzodiazepines) (Table 1.3). Whether these drugs offer some prophylactic advantage or, on the contrary, predispose to NMS cannot be answered as yet based on the limited and uncontrolled data now available. However, evidence derived from cases of neuroleptic-related heatstroke (Chapter 2) strongly suggests a contributory role of anticholinergics in impairing heat loss, such that administration of anticholinergics may be disadvantageous in patients with high temperature in NMS.

Although NMS may occur acutely, for example, after an overdose of neuroleptics (Klein et al. 1985), it typically develops over 1 to 3 days. Two-thirds of cases develop by 1 week, and 96 percent within 30 days of drug exposure (Caroff and Mann 1988). This suggests that although mechanisms underlying NMS appear to be related to early phases of treatment, NMS is not necessarily a fulminant reaction. Furthermore, variability in time of onset indicates that factors other than neuroleptic treatment per se are relevant in triggering NMS and potentially could serve as predictive risk factors.

TABLE 1.3. Concurrent Drugs Associated With 219 NMS Episodes

Drug	N	%
Antiparkinsonian drugs	55	25
Lithium (0.9 ± 0.4 mEq/l)	35	16
TCA	16	7
Benzodiazepines	10	5

Clinical Variables

Unfortunately, aside from a history of previous NMS episodes and the fact that males outnumber females by about two to one among reported cases, the occurrence of NMS remains essentially idiosyncratic. It has been suggested that young adult males (Caroff 1980), children (Klein et al. 1985; Moore et al. 1986; Shields and Bray 1976) and adolescents (Geller and Greydanus 1979) are at increased risk for NMS. However, all ages have been affected (Figure 1.1), and the age-related incidence may simply parallel neuroleptic usage.

Patients treated with neuroleptics for psychosis associated with mood disorders (Addonizio et al. 1986; Pearlman 1986) or preexisting brain disease (Caroff 1980; Delay and Deniker 1968; Vincent et al. 1986) may be more susceptible to NMS, although patients with a range of psychiatric disorders and even presumptive normal individuals exposed to neuroleptics may develop NMS (Moyes 1973; Patel and Bristow 1987) (Table 1.4). However, except for the prevalence of mood disorders among patients with NMS, which appears to be greater than that expected from the usual distribution of diagnoses of patients treated with neuroleptics, NMS is not specific to any diagnostic category.

Alcoholic patients may have a lower threshold of resistance to neurotoxic side effects of antipsychotic drugs (Lutz 1976), and hence may be more susceptible to NMS. Alcoholism was diagnosed in 8 percent of NMS patients in one review (Levenson 1985). A particularly vulnerable time to develop NMS may be during acute withdrawal from alcohol or CNS depressant drugs (Burch and Downs 1987; George and Woods 1987; Greenblatt et al. 1978), when neurologic status and thermoregulatory and autonomic mechanisms are already compromised.

That the physiological state of the patient may figure prominently in the development of NMS is supported by additional observations. For example, Itoh et al. (1977) found that physical exhaustion and dehydration preceded the onset of NMS in all 14 patients in their series. Harsh (1987) found relative dehydration before the onset of NMS in eight of nine patients.

Van Putten (1974) reported that approximately 20 percent of chronic schizophrenic patients on maintenance antipsychotic drug therapy may experience a change in the "extrapyramidal threshold" over time, sometimes suddenly. McEvoy (1986) observed that improvement in psychotic symptoms may be accompanied by the occurrence of

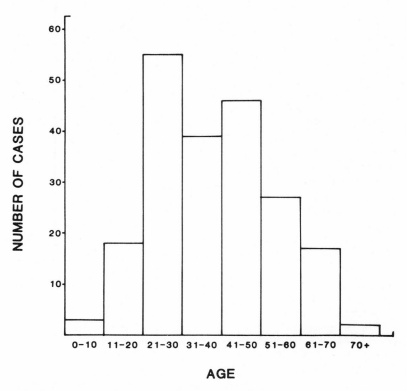

FIGURE 1.1. Age distribution of 206 reported NMS cases.

13

distressing extrapyramidal symptoms, requiring lowered doses of maintenance neuroleptics. He speculated that important changes in neuronal physiology may underlie rapid shifts in both therapeutic and extrapyramidal effects of neuroleptics.

Primeau et al. (1987) postulated that poorly controlled extrapyramidal symptoms in neuroleptic-treated patients may be a risk factor for NMS. They reported that a change to a lesser anticholinergic drug (diphenhydramine) apparently precipitated NMS in three patients receiving haloperidol. In a similar report (Merriam 1987), NMS was precipitated by the apparent loss of cholinergic blockade consequent to a reduction in imipramine dose. Kuehnle (1983) felt that the emergence of neuroleptic-induced dystonic reactions in patients prophylactically treated with anticholinergics may warn of impending NMS. These reports suggest that more active attempts to control or prevent extrapyramidal symptoms by using antiparkinsonian drugs may be beneficial in preventing NMS, as suggested by Levinson and Simpson (1986). However, particularly in view of clinical data showing a failure of antiparkinsonian anticholinergics to prevent or treat symptoms of NMS, it is possible that resistant extrapyramidal symptoms may herald NMS and could indicate the need for recognition and management of NMS.

TABLE 1.4. Underlying Diagnoses Reported in 195 NMS Cases

Diagnosis	N	%
Schizophrenia	66	34
Affective disorder	62	32
Organic brain syndrome (DTs, dementia, post-op, etc.)	25	13
Other neuropsychiatric diagnosis (atypical psychosis, anxiety, etc.)	19	10
Mental retardation	12	6
Schizoaffective disorder	7	4
No neuropsychiatric diagnosis	4	2

Interestingly, an NMS-like syndrome has been reported in association with various extrapyramidal disorders, including Parkinson's disease (see Chapter 3), Huntington's disease (Burke et al. 1981), Wilson's disease (Kontaxakis et al. 1988), striatonigral degeneration (Gibb 1988), and tardive dyskinesia/dystonia (Haggerty et al. 1987; Harris et al. 1987), suggesting that patients with preexisting dysfunction of central dopamine systems may be more susceptible to NMS. A relative imbalance between dopaminergic and cholinergic systems may be a critical determinant in the development of NMS in such cases.

Environmental Factors

Most cases of NMS have been reported from the United States and continental Europe, but the syndrome has also been described in publications from Canada, Great Britain, Ireland, Australia, South Africa, India, Israel, and Japan, as well as other countries. The worldwide occurrence of NMS suggests that environmental factors do not play a primary role in causing the syndrome. Although Singh (1984) claimed there were more frequent reports of NMS from countries with hot climates, based on the author's experience with a case that may have been heatstroke rather than NMS, NMS has occurred with ambient temperatures as low as 8.5 °C (Schroder 1982). Moreover, recent analyses (Caroff and Mann 1988; Shalev et al. 1986) of the occurrence of NMS cases by month demonstrated that NMS was not associated with hot summer months and that it occurred throughout the seasons (Figure 1.2). However, this does not preclude the possibility that hot weather may trigger episodes of NMS in some instances (Shalev et al. 1988).

Clinical and Laboratory Features

Patients with classic signs of NMS present in "hypothalamic" or "adrenergic" crisis, with evidence of increased oxygen utilization (May et al. 1983). Rigidity, unresponsive to anticholinergic treatment, or muscle hypertonicity is often the first presenting sign. Additional parkinsonian features such as tremor, sialorrhea, hypomimia, bradykinesia, and festinating gait may be present. Tremors are frequent, generalized, symmetrical, and impressive. Other neurologic dysfunction may include dystonia, chorea, trismus, dyskinesia, opisthotonos, oculogyric crises, opsoclonus, blepharospasm, dysarthria, dysphagia, abnormal reflexes and posturing, nystagmus, ocular flutter, and seizures (Kurlan et al. 1984). NMS may occur without evidence of severe extrapyramidal symptoms if patients are simultaneously taking muscle relaxants (Rodgers and Stoudemire 1988).

Hyperthermia usually develops concomitantly with or shortly after rigidity. Body temperature has exceeded 40 °C

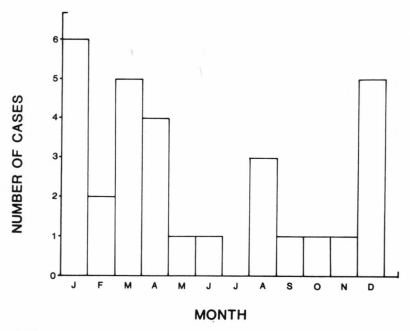

FIGURE 1.2. Seasonality of 30 NMS cases.

in about 40 percent of cases (Addonizio et al. 1987; Caroff and Mann 1988), and temperatures in excess of the 42 °C limit of conventional thermometers have been reported (Bernstein 1979). Hyperthermia is considered by many to be the most distinguishing feature of NMS, setting it apart from other neuroleptic-related conditions with varying combinations of extrapyramidal, autonomic, and neuropsychiatric dysfunction (Fogel and Goldberg 1985). Possible sources of hyperthermia in NMS include neuroleptic-induced inhibition of central dopaminergic thermoregulatory mechanisms mediating heat loss, and increased heat production derived from neuroleptic effects on skeletal muscle tone and metabolism. Febrile medical complications of NMS—such as infection, dehydration, electrolyte imbalance, pulmonary embolus, atelectasis, rhabdomyolysis, and seizures—may secondarily contribute to elevated temperatures (Levinson and Simpson 1986), but do not explain the development of hyperthermia in most cases (Addonizio et al. 1987; Caroff and Mann 1988).

The patient usually has a diminished awareness of the environment, with a fixed gaze resembling akinetic mutism or locked-in syndrome. Some patients, however, may be agitated, psychotic, and delirious. The level of consciousness may progress from stupor to coma. It is important to differentiate the clinical features of NMS from those of functional decompensation because the clinical condition will surely be aggravated by continued or increased antipsychotic treatment in NMS.

TABLE 1.5. Clinical Manifestations of Reported NMS Cases

Symptom	N	+	%
Temperature			
> 37 C	194	190	98
> 40 C		76	39
Muscle rigidity	187	181	97
Change in mental status	167	164	98
Autonomic dysfunction	153	146	95

17

The autonomic nervous system disturbances in NMS—tachycardia, tachypnea, profuse diaphoresis, labile blood pressure, urinary incontinence, and pallor—may be seen at any time and may provide an early clue to recognizing NMS (Bernstein 1979; Zubenko and Pope 1983). A history of unexplained hyperthermia or autonomic instability during previous treatment with neuroleptics may help identify individuals predisposed to NMS (Haggerty et al. 1987).

While heterogeneity exists among descriptions contained in the numerous case reports in the literature (Levinson and Simpson 1986), in a recent review of 256 NMS cases reported between 1980 and 1987, we found a striking consistency in the findings of hyperthermia, muscle rigidity, changes in mental status, and autonomic dysfunction (Caroff and Mann 1988) (Table 1.5).

Laboratory Findings

Clinical laboratory abnormalities are common in NMS (Table 1.6), but most are nonspecific or reflect complications of the syndrome. Nevertheless, a comprehensive laboratory investigation is essential to rule out other causes of hyperthermia.

The white blood cell count may be elevated to 30,000/mm³ with or without a left shift. Rhabdomyolysis (myonecrosis of skeletal muscle cells) may result in markedly increased levels of serum CPK and visible myoglobinuria (i.e., dark brown, orthotolidine-positive urine without red cells). CPK

TABLE 1.6. Positive Laboratory Findings Reported in NMS Cases

Examination	N	+	%	Comments
Creatine phosphokinase (mm)	140	133	95	1–2000X
Myoglobin	30	20	67	
White blood count	107	105	98	up to 35,000
Arterial blood gas	20	15	75	
Electroencephalogram	65	35	54	

elevations may occur in up to 95 percent of NMS cases (Caroff and Mann 1988), reaching as high as 2,000 times normal values in some cases. More commonly, modest or equivocal elevations occur, which cannot be distinguished from the effects of nonspecific factors (e.g., agitation and elevated body temperature). Serum aldolase may also be elevated, along with other serum enzymes (transaminases, lactic dehydrogenase), which may reflect damage to the liver and other tissues.

Arterial blood-gas abnormalities are common and usually reflect metabolic acidosis and hypoxia. Findings indicative of disseminated intravascular coagulation—such as increased prothrombin time and activated partial thromboplastin time, increased fibrin split products, and decreased platelets—have been reported in several cases (Allsop and Twigley 1987; Eles et al. 1984; Martin et al. 1985; Surmont 1981; Yasukawa et al. 1983). Cases of NMS have been reported in association with both hyponatremia (Gibb et al. 1986; Tomson 1986; Wedzicha and Hoffbrand 1984) and hypernatremia (Chayasirisobhon et al. 1983; Ewert et al. 1983; Klein et al. 1985). These alterations in sodium may not have significance apart from the profound fluid and electrolyte disturbances that may develop in NMS, although some investigators have proposed hyponatremia or inappropriate antidiuretic hormone secretion as precipitating factors in NMS (Gibb et al. 1986; Tomson 1986).

In 75 cases reported between 1980 and 1987 in which the results of evaluation for sepsis were specified, multiple cultures of body fluids failed to identify an organism that could account for the syndrome (Caroff and Mann 1988) (Table 1.7). Thus most reported cases of NMS are not

TABLE 1.7. Negative Laboratory Findings Reported in NMS Cases

Examination	N	− %	
Computed tomography	56	53	95
Cerebrospinal fluid	77	73	95
Cultures (blood, urine, cerebrospinal fluid)	75	75	100

infectious in origin. However, cultures may be positive in cases secondarily complicated by infection (Sherman et al. 1983).

Electroencephalographic examination may be abnormal in about 50 percent of NMS cases, revealing generalized, nonspecific slowing consistent with encephalopathy in most instances. Normal computerized tomographic scans of the head have been obtained in 95 percent of cases reported in the literature (Caroff and Mann 1988). The few abnormal scans revealed evidence of preexisting pathology (e.g., atrophy or trauma). Similarly, examination of cerebrospinal fluid (CSF) was normal in 95 percent of cases (Caroff and Mann 1988). These results suggest that it is unlikely that a central organic etiology, unrelated to drug treatment, is responsible for the clinical manifestations of NMS in most cases.

Increased peripheral levels of monoamines and their metabolites have been reported in NMS and undoubtedly reflect the autonomic activation or "adrenergic crisis" that occurs as part of NMS (Feibel and Schiffer 1981; Hashimoto et al. 1984). In several cases, monoamine metabolites were measured in CSF to assess neurotransmitter activity in the brain (Table 1.8). Ansseau et al. (1980) found increased homovanillic acid (HVA) and normal 5-hydroxyindoleacetic

TABLE 1.8. Measurements of CSF Monoamine Metabolites Reported in NMS Cases

Reference	Methodology	HVA	5-HIAA
Ansseau et al. (1980)	———	Increased	Normal
Granato et al. (1983)	HPLC	Normal	———
Tollefson and Garvey (1984)	LC	Increased	Increased
Pirovino et al. (1984)	HPLC	Normal	Normal
Verhoeven et al. (1985)	HPLC	Decreased	———
Ansseau et al. (1986)	GC	Increased	Normal

Note. HVA = homovanillic acid; 5-HIAA = 5-hydroxyindoleacetic acid; HPLC = high performance liquid chromatography; LC = liquid chromatography; GC = gas chromatography.

20

acid (5-HIAA) in one patient. Granato et al. (1983) reported a normal level of HVA that decreased within the normal range in correlation with clinical improvement following treatment with bromocriptine. Pirovino et al. (1984) found normal levels of CSF metabolites. Tollefson and Garvey (1984) found elevations of 3,4-dihydroxyphenylacetic acid, HVA, and 5-HIAA in an NMS case. In another patient with NMS, Verhoeven et al. (1985) found slightly lowered HVA, whereas Ansseau et al. (1986) reported slightly elevated HVA and normal 5-HIAA; Yamawaki (1986) found the opposite in a patient treated with amitriptyline. Thus there has been no consistent pattern of neurotransmitter metabolites in the CSF of patients with NMS studied to date. However, data are limited to individual case reports in which differing laboratory techniques are used to measure metabolites and in which critical comparisons with appropriate control groups, such as normal individuals and neuroleptic-treated and untreated schizophrenic patients, are lacking. Interpretation of these data would be premature until further controlled studies are conducted.

Abnormal in vitro skeletal muscle contracture responses to halothane may occur, similar to those seen in patients with malignant hyperthermia (Araki et al. 1988; Caroff et al. 1987a; Denborough et al. 1984). These data appear to correlate with clinical similarities between NMS and malignant hyperthermia. However, contrary reports exist (Krivosic-Horber et al. 1987; Merry et al. 1986; Tollefson and Garvey 1984), and the contracture test itself remains controversial, leaving unresolved the issue of in vitro muscle biopsy testing as a potential marker for NMS. Muscle histopathology has been normal or revealed only nonspecific changes (Araki et al. 1988; Heiman-Patterson et al., unpublished data; Scarlett et al. 1983; Surmont et al. 1984). Studies on muscle pathophysiology in NMS are reviewed in more detail in Chapter 4.

We found autopsy data reported in 20 fatal cases of NMS. There were no abnormal CNS findings in five cases (Henry et al. 1971; Itoh et al. 1977; Kinross-Wright 1958;

Morris et al. 1980). In three cases there was no other specific pathology that could account for the cause of death (Merriam 1987; Moyes 1973; Straker 1986). Postmortem findings in the remaining cases revealed abnormalities of the brain and viscera generally believed to be the result of hyperthermia, medical complications or unrelated disorders (Ansseau et al. 1986; Eiser et al. 1982; Klein et al. 1985; Prunier and Frankel 1986; Regestein et al. 1977; Surmont et al. 1984; Ungvari 1987; Brennan et al. 1988; Horn et al. 1988; McCarthy et al. 1988). For example, "atypical" brain lesions were observed in three cases of NMS, probably due to the effects of hyperthermia and/or hypoxia rather than a direct effect of the neuroleptic (Surmont et al. 1984). Likewise, Horn et al. (1988) reported a fatal case of NMS associated with hypothalamic lesions "similar in nature and distribution to those anoxia-ischemia" (p. 619). This underscores the difficulty in interpreting postmortem findings in NMS since changes may occur secondarily and may not be related directly to the underlying pathophysiological mechanisms.

Diagnosis

Although there is currently no formal consensus as to what constellation of signs and symptoms constitute the NMS, a number of investigators have proposed diagnostic criteria. Levenson (1985) suggested that the presence of three major manifestations (fever, rigidity, and increased CPK) or two major and four of six minor manifestations (tachycardia, abnormal blood pressure, tachypnea, altered consciousness, diaphoresis, and leukocytosis) indicated a high probability of NMS if supported by the clinical history.

However, this formulation was criticized by Roth and associates (1986) for several reasons. First, it permits the diagnosis of NMS in the absence of muscular rigidity, and therefore does not adequately delineate NMS from heat-stroke, which usually presents with flaccid muscles. Second, increased levels of CPK in psychiatric patients may be caused by many conditions other than NMS: muscle trauma, struggling against restraints, dystonic reactions, and intramuscular injections. Acute psychosis alone has been associated with increased CPK levels in hospitalized patients (Coryell et al. 1978; Meltzer et al. 1980), although usually not to the degree observed in some NMS cases. Third, Roth et al. (1986) found CPK elevations in only three of eight patients who may have developed a "milder, self-limited form of neuroleptic malignant syndrome" (p. 673), far below the 97 percent of patients reported by Levenson (1985) and the 95 percent reported by Caroff and Mann (1988).

Points raised by Roth et al. (1986) underscore the difficulties in developing criteria for NMS since most of the individual symptoms are nonspecific and can be caused by factors other than neuroleptics (Chapters 3 and 5). However, there is a surprising consistency in the identification of the major clinical features of NMS in reported cases. This de facto consensus is reflected in diagnostic criteria proposed by other authors (Addonizio et al. 1986; Pope et al. 1986b). Pope et al. (1986b) suggested that NMS was diagnosable based on hyperthermia, severe extrapyramidal symptoms, and autonomic dysfunction, and that altered mental status, leukocytosis, and elevated CPK could be used retrospectively to support the diagnosis. Similarly, Addonizio et al. (1986) proposed that elevated temperature, extrapyramidal symptoms, and a combination of autonomic signs, confusion, and laboratory values could be used to support the diagnosis.

Apart from minor variations, these sets of criteria are quite similar, particularly in the recognition that hyperthermia and muscle rigidity are cardinal features of NMS. Consistent with previously proposed criteria, we suggest that definite diagnostic criteria for NMS include the concurrent development of hyperthermia, muscle rigidity, and a combination of mental status and autonomic and laboratory abnormalities in patients receiving or recently treated with neuroleptics (Table 1.9). In addition, criteria should stipulate that systemic or neuropsychiatric causes of NMS-like disorders have been excluded. The reliability and clinical significance of these criteria could be tested in future investigations.

Probable or possible NMS cases reported as "atypical" (Bernstein 1979; Misiaszek and Potter 1985) or "paradoxical" (Price and Giannini 1983), in which the full constellation of signs and symptoms (fever, rigidity, autonomic disturbances, and altered mental status) are not present, remain controversial. In such *formes frustes*, either rigidity or hyperthermia did not develop. Whether these instances represent abortive cases of NMS that were detected early, before the full-blown syndrome developed, and then treated promptly, (Clark et al. 1986; Grey 1986), or whether these cases fall along a continuum of neuroleptic toxicity of less severity than NMS (Brown et al. 1986; Conlon 1986; Fogel and Goldberg 1985) remains unclear. Addonizio and colleagues (1986) favored the latter explanation in view of their finding that symptoms in these cases sometimes abate without cessation of neuroleptic treatment. Similarly, Brown et al. (1986) proposed that NMS-like reactions represented a continuum, based on the degree and the central sites of dopamine blockade. On the

TABLE 1.9. Proposed Diagnostic Criteria for NMS

1. Treatment with neuroleptics within 7 days prior to onset
   (4 weeks for depot drugs)
2. Hyperthermia ($\geq$ 38° C)
3. Muscle rigidity
4. Three of the following:

   a. change in mental status
   b. tachycardia
   c. hypertension or hypotension
   d. tachypnea or hypoxia
   e. creatine phosphokinase elevation or myoglobinuria
   f. leukocytosis
   g. metabolic acidosis

5. Not due to systemic or neuropsychiatric illness

Note. All five items required concurrently.

other hand, Adityanjee et al. (1988) felt that the spectrum concept was an "artifact" based on the "arbitrary" nature by which NMS is defined and diagnosed (p. 110).

Ambiguity surrounding the diagnosis of NMS also stems from the fact that some cases reported as NMS were actually unrelated to treatment with neuroleptics (see Chapter 3). Examples of "nonneuroleptic" malignant syndrome (Cohen et al. 1987) include the use of dopamine-depleting agents in a patient with Huntington's disease (Burke et al. 1981), and treatment with tricyclic antidepressants alone (Burch and Downs 1987; Grant 1984; Lesaca 1987; Taylor and Schwartz 1988) and in combination with monoamine oxidase inhibitors (Ritchie 1983). Other cases labeled NMS followed withdrawal of dopamine-potentiating drugs in patients with Parkinson's disease (see Chapter 3), Alzheimer's disease (Rosse and Ciolino 1985), and schizophrenia (Lazarus 1985b). One report described a syndrome identical to NMS in a patient treated with phenelzine, lorazepam, and atenolol but not with neuroleptics (Cohen et al. 1987). Phenelzine in combination with lithium carbonate, L–tryptophan, diazepam, and triazolam, has also been reported to produce an NMS-like syndrome (Brennan et al. 1988).

Straker (1986) suggested the appellation "hypo-dopaminergic malignant syndrome" for NMS-like states due to central dopamine depletion caused by nonneuroleptic agents. Whether these are bona fide cases of NMS or similar drug-induced subtypes of a more generalized *syndrome malin* that may occur in susceptible patients due to various pharmacologic agents remains uncertain (Caroff 1980). To avoid confusion, Lazarus (1985c) recommended reserving use of the term *neuroleptic malignant syndrome* for those cases caused primarily by neuroleptic administration.

Inconsistency in the definition and boundaries of NMS has become a major source of criticism that has led some clinicians to consider the term *neuroleptic malignant syndrome* "unnecessary and possibly alarmist" (p. 129) (Clough

25

1983). Others have been moved to abolish use of the term altogether, citing the potential for confusion and misapplication (Levinson and Simpson 1986). There is concern that some conditions are incorrectly being diagnosed as NMS, that infatuation with NMS may divert attention from treating medically ill febrile patients, or that the diagnosis of NMS will cause clinicians to withhold neuroleptics from chronic schizophrenic patients who require long-term therapy and yet might not develop the syndrome on repeated exposure to neuroleptics.

Although all of these concerns merit consideration, and it is conceivable that patients labeled as having NMS might have medical explanations for their disorder (Levinson and Simpson 1986), in practice the diagnosis of NMS is usually made by exclusion after puzzled clinicians have ruled out or treated all medical factors (Caroff et al. 1987b; Ingraham et al. 1982). Rarely has a case been reported where another condition was overlooked or mismanaged because NMS was considered instead. The syndrome is more apt to be missed or not entertained at all, and patients with NMS may be neglected or receive improper treatment.

Levenson (1986) pointed out that it is often difficult to determine whether coincident medical conditions represent complications or alternative diagnoses, yet this hardly seems sufficient reason to abandon use of the term *neuroleptic malignant syndrome*. Unquestionably, the term has provocative connotations, and its historical derivation is obscure to most clinicians, yet it underscores the need for recognizing the role of neuroleptics in causing extrapyramidal symptoms with hyperthermia when other potential causes have been eliminated. In cases of diagnostic uncertainty, "it is less useful to focus on whether or not the patient has NMS than to determine what should be done therapeutically" (p. 1292) (Fogel and Goldberg 1985), that is, discontinue neuroleptics and undertake a rigorous evaluation until a specific etiology is found or symptoms resolve (Caroff 1980).

TABLE 1.10. Medical Illnesses Resembling NMS

Neurological Disorders
    Meningitis
    Viral encephalitis
    Neurosyphilis
    Parkinson's disease
    Wilson's disease
    Cerebrovascular disease
    Head trauma
    Epilepsy
    Myotonia
    Akinetic mutism
    Stiff man syndrome
    Locked-in syndrome
Metabolic and Endocrine Disorders
    Hepatic encephalopathy
    Acute intermittent porphyria
    Hypocalcemia (tetany)
    Thyrotoxicosis (thyroid storm)
    Diabetic ketoacidosis
    Pheochromocytoma
    Myxedema
    Addison's disease
Toxins
    Tetanus
    Strychnine
    Curare
    Botulism
    MPTP
    Phencyclidine
Psychotropic-Drug Related Conditions
    Neuroleptic-induced catatonia
    MAO inhibitor-tricyclic antidepressant combinations
    Sedative-hypnotic withdrawal
    Stimulant abuse
    Anticholinergic toxicity
Disorders of Temperature Regulation
    Malignant hyperthermia
    Heatstroke
Miscellaneous
    Remote effects of carcinoma
    Collagen-vascular disorders (lupus, polymyositis)

Note. Adapted from Lazarus (1985), with permission.

Differential Diagnosis

NMS may present a baffling array of disturbances mimicking neurologic, infectious, vascular, neoplastic, or toxic-metabolic diseases (Table 1.10). The diagnosis may be obscured by seemingly inconsistent physical findings such as pallor in the presence of hyperthermia and hypertension consequent to antipsychotic drug therapy. NMS should be considered in any febrile patient receiving neuroleptics, especially if there are concomitant extrapyramidal side effects. On the other hand, it would be erroneous, if not harmful, to diagnose NMS to the exclusion of various medical illnesses that may simulate NMS.

Many medical disorders may simulate NMS by causing catatonia and mutism (Altshuler et al. 1986; Gelenberg 1976; Mann et al. 1986). Neurologic conditions to be considered include idiopathic and arteriosclerotic parkinsonism, herpetic or epidemic encephalitis, neurosyphilis, traumatic hemorrhage in the region of the third ventricle, focal lesions of the thalamus and frontal lobe, closed head injury, Wernicke's encephalopathy, tuberous sclerosis, the postictal phase of epilepsy, and others. Metabolic derangements such as diabetic ketoacidosis, hypocalcemia (tetany), and acute intermittent porphyria may cause catatonic symptoms, with or without mutism. When catatonia is associated with marked autonomic disturbances, thyrotoxicosis, pheochromocytoma, and hyperdynamic beta-adrenergic circulatory state should be considered (Ries and Schuckit 1980). Other possible disorders simulating NMS include lupus cerebritis and remote effects of carcinoma.

Toxic agents may cause rigidity and catatonia or hyperthermia and may resemble NMS. Organic fluorides, tetanus, strychnine, curare, and botulism are examples. Reactions to other psychotropic drugs—including tricyclic antidepressants, monoamine oxidase inhibitors, stimulants, and hallucinogens—should be considered in the differential diagnosis of NMS, as discussed in Chapter 3.

Withdrawal from alcohol and sedative-hypnotic drugs can lead to thermoregulatory and autonomic dysfunction, but this is not usually confused with NMS. However, a picture consistent with NMS has been reported in patients treated with neuroleptics during withdrawal (Burch and Downs 1987; George and Wood 1987; Greenblatt et al. 1978), suggesting that neuroleptics should be used cautiously in these patients.

Although NMS may represent the more severe and hyperacute end of the spectrum of extrapyramidal disorders due to neuroleptics, its potential for morbidity and special treatment considerations suggest that it should be recognized apart from more benign neuroleptic-related conditions. For example, intercurrent infections and fever may develop in the context of neuroleptic-induced extrapyramidal symptoms, but this differs from NMS in clinical and laboratory findings, correlation with neuroleptic use, and response to specific drugs (e.g., antibiotics and antiparkinsonian anticholinergic drugs vs. bromocriptine and dantrolene). Moreover, patients with neuroleptic-induced catatonia do not exhibit the severe hyperthermia and autonomic dysregulation found in NMS (Stoudemire and Luther 1984).

The similarities between NMS, heatstroke, malignant hyperthermia, and lethal catatonia have led to speculation about their association. Table 1.11 presents similar and contrasting findings in NMS and these three conditions, which are described more fully in the following chapters. All are characterized by the presence of hyperthermia associated with abnormal vital signs and various metabolic derangements, often leading in the extreme form to acidosis, myoglobinuria, renal failure, coagulation abnormalities, coma, and death. Muscle rigidity and diaphoresis are common in all conditions except heatstroke, which usually presents with dry skin and decreased muscle tone. Although neuroleptics increase the risk of heatstroke (Kilbourne et al. 1982), environmental exposure and/or strenuous activity are the primary causes, whereas NMS usually occurs independent of these factors.

Malignant hyperthermia, which appears to have a genetic basis in most cases, is rapid in onset and occurs in a perioperative setting following use of inhalational or muscle-depolarizing anesthetics. The clinical differentiation of malignant hyperthermia from NMS may present a dilemma in the postoperative patient treated with neuroleptics (Kuhn and Lippmann 1987) (see Chapter 4).

Lethal catatonia probably represents a nonspecific syndrome, which may develop during a variety of organic as well as functional illnesses (Mann et al. 1986). Based on this definition, NMS may be conceptualized as a neuroleptic-induced or iatrogenic form of organic lethal catatonia. Thus the diagnostic evaluation of a suspected NMS episode involves the exclusion of other causes of lethal catatonia. While it is difficult to distinguish NMS from lethal catatonia due to other causes, neuroleptic drugs should be discontinued in either case because they may be hazardous in NMS and

TABLE 1.11. Comparison of NMS, Malignant Hyperthermia, Heatstroke, and Lethal Catatonia

	NMS	Malignant Hyperthermia	Heatstroke	Lethal Catatonia (functional origin)
Hyperthermia	yes	yes	yes	yes
Muscle rigidity	yes	yes	not typical	yes
Diaphoresis	yes	yes	not typical	yes
Tachycardia	yes	yes	yes	yes
Acidosis	yes	yes	yes	?
Coagulopathy	yes	yes	yes	?
Myoglobinuria	yes	yes	yes	?
Mental status	impaired	impaired	impaired	impaired
Genetic predisposition	no	often	no	no
Precipitant	neuroleptics	halothane, succinylcholine, ? stress	exposure or exercise	?
Onset	hours–days	minutes–hours	minutes–hours	days–weeks
Mortality	10–20%	30%	20–50%	75–100%
Therapy	dantrolene, dopaminergic agonists	dantrolene	? dantrolene	ECT, corticosteroids

ineffective in advanced stages of lethal catatonia regardless of etiology (see Chapter 5).

A complete medical and psychiatric history and careful neurologic and physical examination is mandatory to differentiate NMS from these various conditions. In addition, the following laboratory studies are recommended: complete blood cell count with differential, erythrocyte sedimentation rate, serum electrolytes, and calcium; kidney, liver, and thyroid function tests; toxicology screen; serologic test for syphilis; antinuclear antibody and lupus erythematosus prep; early determination of serum CPK levels; urinalysis for myoglobinuria; lumbar puncture; electroencephalogram; and computerized tomography or magnetic resonance imaging of the brain. Diseases that resemble NMS often reveal specific laboratory abnormalities not found in NMS, whereas in NMS there are no pathognomonic findings.

It should be kept in mind that NMS can affect nonpsychiatric patients treated with phenothiazines and other dopamine-blocking agents used for nausea and vomiting (Moore et al. 1986; Preston 1959; Robinson et al. 1985; Samie 1987), agitation (Cahill and Arana 1986; Kuhn and Lippmann 1987; Vincent et al. 1986), chronic pain (Prunier and Frankel 1986), and other purposes (Chayasirisobhon et al. 1983; Moyes 1973). Because a psychiatric disorder is not a prerequisite for developing NMS, a high index of suspicion is usually required to make the diagnosis when these drugs are employed.

Complications

Many patients with NMS sustain significant morbidity during the course of their illness. Diverse complications involving cardiac, respiratory, renal, musculoskeletal, and other systems may be seen. More than one-third of patients have required treatment in an intensive care setting (Lavie et al. 1986a). This was the case with a 36-year-old woman who suffered an acute myocardial infarction with pulmonary edema (Bernstein 1979), and a 64-year-old man who developed a cardiac arrhythmia, followed by a seizure, cardiac arrest, and dysphagia persisting for 2 months, leading to aspiration pneumonia (Cruz et al. 1983). In one case of NMS complicated by infection with gas producing *Escherichia coli*, the patient required bilateral below-the-knee fasciotomies (Sherman et al. 1983).

Myoglobinuric renal failure consequent to rhabdomyolysis is one of the more common and more serious complications of NMS (Eiser et al. 1982), occurring in 16 to 25 percent of cases (Levenson 1985; Shalev and Munitz 1986). The precise mechanism by which myoglobinuria causes acute renal failure is unknown. Possibilities include renal tubular obstruction due to myoglobin precipitation within the tubular lumen, and acute tubular necrosis resulting from ischemia (decreased renal blood flow and glomerular filtration rate) or myoglobin nephrotoxicity (Knochel 1981). The development of a red or brown color in the urine should immediately signal the possibility of myoglobinuria so that appropriate therapy with hydration, diuretics, and osmotic agents can be given. Dialysis will be required if renal insufficiency ensues, but dialysis will not remove the offending neuroleptic from serum because neuroleptics are highly membrane or protein bound.

It is important to recognize that myoglobinuria has a wide variety of etiologies and may not be as rare as previously thought. The cause of myoglobinuria in NMS is probably multifactorial: immobilization; intramuscular injections; muscle necrosis due to severe rigidity, catatonic posturing, or coma; hyperthermia; and dehydration. Myoglobinuria may be seen in psychiatric patients with neuroleptic-related conditions other than NMS, for example, in neuroleptic-induced dystonic reactions (Cavanaugh and Finlayson 1984; Ravi et al. 1982), rapid intramuscular "neuroleptization" (Thase and Shostak 1984), and (rarely) in tardive dyskinesia (Lazarus and Toglia 1985).

Psychiatric patients in particular appear to be at high risk for developing rhabdomyolysis and renal failure (Johnson et al. 1987; Lazarus 1985d). Psychotropic agents alone may cause rhabdomyolysis (Abreo et al. 1982; Johnson et al. 1986), but most case reports involve other factors: abnormal movements, repeated intramuscular injections, exertion against restraints (often in conjunction with drug or alcohol intoxication), or erratic oral intake (Johnson et al. 1987). Occasionally, behavioral disturbances in psychiatric patients predispose them to rhabdomyolysis (Coryell et al. 1978; Finlayson and Cavanaugh 1985). Recognizing psychiatric patients who may be at higher risk for developing this muscle problem is important because early detection and timely therapy may reduce morbidity and mortality (e.g., from renal failure) in many instances.

Respiratory distress is another frequent complication of NMS. Levenson (1985) observed that ventilator support was necessary for 10 of 53 patients with NMS. Respiratory failure in NMS may be caused by aspiration due to impaired deglutition, infection, shock, pulmonary emboli, neuroleptic-induced decreased chest wall compliance, and necrosis of respiratory muscles due to rhabdomyolysis. The normal size and configuration of the cardiac silhouette on chest X ray suggests that pulmonary edema in NMS is noncardiogenic (Martin et al. 1985).

Although Delay and Deniker (1968) originally considered respiratory abnormalities an integral part of the NMS symptom complex, other authors believed that acute respiratory insufficiency in neuroleptic-treated patients constituted a separate entity (Auzépy et al. 1977; Giroud et al. 1978). However, a review (Buffat et al. 1985) of this controversy did not support the distinction. Most patients who developed respiratory insufficiency while on neuroleptics also showed features common to NMS: extrapyramidal rigidity, hyperthermia, rhabdomyolysis, and a favorable response to dantrolene. It may be that in some patients with NMS, severe respiratory abnormalities predominate; these patients may be predisposed to pulmonary problems on the basis of chronic obstructive pulmonary disease or a preexisting immune deficiency (Buffat et al. 1985).

Persistent neuromuscular abnormalities have been reported in several patients with NMS. Residual muscle stiffness is not uncommon (Bates and Courtenay-Evans 1984; Jessee and Anderson 1983; Lazarus, 1985c). Rigidity may be severe enough to cause joint subluxation, muscle avulsion, and contractures of the extremities (Mueller 1985). Other neurologic impairments may include permanent dystonia (Mueller et al. 1983) and polyneuropathy (Anderson and Weinschenk 1987; Eiser et al. 1982) resulting in weakness and sensory impairment. Brain damage and permanent coma was reported in one case of NMS following ECT and cardiac arrest (Regestein et al. 1987).

Cases of NMS involving the coadministration of lithium or complicated by severe hyperthermia may result in cortical and cerebellar damage with cognitive impairment, neuropsychiatric abnormalities, persistent ataxia, dyskinesias, dysarthria, and apraxia (Bond et al. 1984; Cohen and Cohen 1974; Lefkowitz et al. 1983; Rothke and Bush 1986). The cerebellum has been shown to be particularly sensitive to the effects of lithium salts, even in therapeutic doses (Apte and Langston 1983; Donaldson and Cunningham 1983). In addition, the cerebellum appears to be extremely sensitive to the effects of hyperthermia (Freeman and Dumoff 1944; Malamud et al. 1946).

Despite therapeutic efforts, 25 (10 percent) of 256 cases of NMS reported between 1980 and 1987 ended in death (Caroff and Mann 1988). However, due to biases in reporting, more accurate estimates of mortality may be derived from series of NMS cases studied by individual groups (Table 1.12). Such reports reveal an apparent decline in the mortality rate of NMS, from 20 to 30 percent in the 1970s (Fabre et al. 1977; Itoh et al. 1977) to no fatalities in original series of patients reported recently (Addonizio et al. 1986; Pearlman 1986). This apparent decline is encouraging and may reflect earlier diagnosis, rapid drug discontinuation and institution of intensive care, or use of specific therapeutic drugs. Nevertheless, NMS remains potentially lethal.

Pathogenesis

Most clinical evidence suggests that impaired dopamine neurotransmission mediated by neuroleptic-induced dopamine receptor blockade is of primary importance in NMS (Henderson and Wooten 1981; Hermesh et al. 1984). This derives from knowledge that while neuroleptics have various actions, blockade of dopamine receptors is common to all (Creese et al. 1983). Also supporting this hypothesis is the observation that various other pharmacologic manipulations appear to cause NMS through reduced dopamine activity. Examples include induction of NMS with nonneuroleptic dopamine-blocking drugs such as metoclopramide (Finucane and Murphy 1984; Robinson et al. 1985; Samie 1987); depletion of dopamine storage pools with alpha-methyltyrosine, tetrabenazine, and reserpine (Burke et al. 1981; Haggerty et al. 1987); withdrawal of dopamine agonist drugs in patients with Parkinson's disease (see Chapter 3); and chronic administration of dextroamphetamine in a patient with narcolepsy followed by therapy with neuroleptics (Chayasirisobhon et al. 1983). Alternatively, therapy with dopamine agonist drugs

TABLE 1.12. Mortality Rate in Reported Series of NMS Cases

Reference	N	Deaths	Rate (%)
Itoh et al. (1977)	14	4	29
Fabre et al. (1977)	7	2	29
Auzépy et al. (1977)	37	6	16
Giroud et al. (1978)	11	4	36
Destée et al. (1980)	31	3	10
Kleinknecht et al. (1982)	6	3	50
Kimsey et al. (1983)	6	1	17
Pope et al. (1986b)	8	1	13
Addonizio et al. (1986)	8	0	0
Pearlman (1986)	10	0	0

has been shown to reverse signs and symptoms of NMS (Lazarus 1986a).

Dopamine blockade in the nigrostriatal pathway has been theorized to cause rigidity and parkinsonism in neuroleptic-treated patients (Marsden and Jenner 1980). The actual mechanism by which this occurs is quite complex and probably involves multiple neuronal pathways connected with the basal ganglia. Penney and Young (1983) discussed the importance of a cortico-striato-pallido-thalamocortical feedback circuit responsible for the production of rigidity:

> The model proposes a positive feedback circuit that travels from the motor cortex through the striatum, medial globus pallidus, and thalamus to return to the cortex. Failure to maintain the integrity of these pathways leads to chorea. Inability to suppress activity of this loop leads to parkinsonism. Cholinergic neurons promote the positive feedback loop. Dopaminergic neurons inhibit the circuit. Thus, cholinergic and antidopaminergic agents [e.g., neuroleptics] relieve chorea and produce parkinsonism, whereas anticholinergic and dopaminergic agents relieve parkinsonism and produce chorea. (p. 88)

Neuroleptic-induced blockade of dopamine receptors in the hypothalamus may lead to autonomic impairment and impairment of central thermoregulation, causing hyperthermia through decreased heat dissipation (Henderson and Wooten 1981). It is well established that dopamine is an important neurotransmitter involved in central thermoregulation and that dopamine agonists have hypothermic actions (Cox 1979) (see Chapter 2). Conversely, dopamine blockade with neuroleptics may be associated with hyperthermia (Borbély and Loepfe-Hinkkanen 1979). Experimental data indicate that inhibition of diencephalospinal dopaminergic neurons with neuroleptics could further contribute to autonomic and motor abnormalities in NMS (Lindvall et al. 1983).

Alteration of dopamine neurotransmission in the brainstem reticular activating system may cause mutism and similar disturbances in arousal (Akhtar and Buckman 1977; Behrman 1972). In animal models, lesions of mesencephalic dopaminergic neurons have been associated with various psychomotor abnormalities, including a behavioral state characterized by akinesia, hypertonicity, and decreased responsiveness (Jones et al. 1973; Robbins et al. 1982). Pathways believed to be involved in a similar state of unresponsiveness in humans (i.e., akinetic mutism) are discussed in Chapter 5.

Results of laboratory and biologic tests performed during the acute or recovery stages of NMS further support an association between neuroleptics and dopamine receptor blockade in NMS. Hashimoto and associates (1984) described a patient with NMS whose clinical improvement was paralleled by decreased neuroleptic levels, decreased prolactin levels, and increased responsiveness to intravenous dopamine hydrochloride. Allan and White (1972) reported a patient with NMS whose improvement coincided with a decline in the concentration of urinary fluphenazine breakdown products. Tollefson and Garvey (1984) found no such correlation in a case of chlorpromazine-induced NMS, but they reported marked elevations of dopamine metabolites, 3,4-dihydroxyphenylacetic acid and HVA in CSF (see Table 1.8). Ansseau and colleagues (1986) found increased levels of CSF HVA and urinary 3-methoxy-4-hydroxyphenylglycol, as well as abnormal growth hormone response after apomorphine and clonidine challenge tests, suggesting that NMS may be related not only to central dopaminergic but also alpha-noradrenergic receptor blockade.

Several other authors have noted the involvement of catecholamines other than dopamine in NMS. Feibel and Schiffer (1981) reported an NMS patient with dramatically elevated urinary and plasma levels of norepinephrine and epinephrine, simulating a pheochromocytoma. In another case, plasma epinephrine and norepinephrine levels were also increased (Hashimoto et al. 1984). Similar findings were reported by Wheeler and colleagues (1985) in a patient who had unexplained episodes of catatonia, hypertension, and tachycardia unrelated to treatment with neuroleptics. Feibel and Schiffer (1981) hypothesized that autonomic instability in NMS was mediated in part by hyperactivity of the sympathoadrenomedullary component of the autonomic nervous system, as evidenced by excessive catecholamine excretion. One review of sudden death in neuroleptic-treated patients suggested that the cause of death may be due to the effects of massive catecholamine discharge on the heart, combined with arrhythmogenic properties of neuroleptics (Ellman 1982).

The possibility that neuroleptics may cause a hyperadrenergic state and hemodynamic instability has led some authors (Ansseau et al. 1980; Schibuk and Schachter 1986) to theorize that NMS results from an excess of norepinephrine relative to dopamine. Maximum depletion of dopamine relative to norepinephrine occurs when antidepressants are prescribed with neuroleptics because most antidepressants act in part to block the reuptake of norepinephrine. Clinically, this suggests that an unusually agitated response to antidepressants, possibly reflected in a rise in catecholamines, may herald the development of NMS or unveil a predisposition for its occurrence in certain patients (Eiser et al. 1982; Schibuk and Schachter 1986).

Complex interactions between the catecholaminergic system and other neurotransmitter systems may account for certain features in NMS not readily explained on the basis of dopamine blockade. Lew and Tollefson (1983) have invoked a theoretical role for a relative dopamine/gamma-aminobutyric acid (GABA) imbalance during NMS. They based their theory on the work of Keller et al. (1976), who showed that diazepam, a GABA-mimetic agent, decreased the rate of striatal dopamine turnover and reversed chlorpromazine- and haloperidol-induced increases in dopamine turnover in the rat. Conversely, in another study, postsynaptic dopamine blockade with haloperidol was followed by decreased GABA content in the striatum and the substantia nigra (Kim and Hassler 1975). Thus a striatonigrostriatal feedback loop between dopamine and GABA may exist, similar to the striatal dopamine/acetylcholine system proposed by Snyder et al. (1974). Recent studies have characterized this feedback loop as consisting of three inhibitory neurons in sequence in which GABA, GABA (or glycine), and dopamine are the putative transmitters (Penney and Young 1983).

In NMS a relative deficiency of GABA may be of primary pathogenic significance or, more likely, may occur secondary to central dopamine blockade. Restoration of the dopamine/GABA balance with GABA-mimetic agents such as diazepam and lorazepam has been therapeutic in some cases of NMS (Fricchione et al. 1983; Lew and Tollefson 1983). Similar improvement has been noted in some patients with Parkinson's disease treated with GABA agonist drugs (Bergmann et al. 1984). On the other hand, high doses of diazepam (100 mg/day or more) caused parkinsonism in 15 percent of schizophrenic patients withdrawn from neuroleptics in one study (Suranyi-Cadotte et al. 1985). Because the relationship between GABA and dopamine is complex—GABA may modulate dopamine-mediated behavior at multiple sites in the CNS (Garbutt and van Kammen 1983)—the relevance of GABAergic mechanisms in NMS must await further clarification.

Sandyk (1985b) has provided evidence supporting the role of the opioid system in the pathogenesis of NMS. Based on experimental studies in laboratory animals, Sandyk (1985b) has proposed that autonomic impairment in NMS represents underactivity, whereas hyperpyrexia and muscular rigidity represent overactivity of the endogenous opioid system. Endogenous opioid peptides appear to modulate the activity of several neurotransmitters at different levels in the

CNS. In the basal ganglia, beta-endorphin modifies the neurotransmission not only of dopamine but also of GABA, substance P, neurotensin, somatostatin, and others (Sandyk 1985a). Injection of beta-endorphin into the CSF of rats may produce prolonged muscular rigidity and immobility similar to a catatonic state, reversed by the opiate antagonist naloxone (Bloom et al. 1976; Wand et al. 1973). However, as Pearlman (1986) pointed out, direct injection of morphine into the substantia nigra pars reticulata and substantia nigra pars compacta has opposite effects on rigidity (Turski et al. 1983), consistent with the observed lack of efficacy of naloxone in NMS (Greenblatt et al. 1978; Irwin and Simon 1984). Furthermore, there is only scant evidence to date implicating endogenous opioid peptides in the control of human motor functions and extrapyramidal disorders (Sandyk 1985a).

In summary, disruption of dopamine neurotransmission in several different dopaminergic tracts, especially those located in the striatum, hypothalamus, brain stem, and spinal cord, appears to account for most of the features in NMS. However, the idiosyncratic occurrence of NMS suggests that factors other than dopamine blockade by neuroleptics are involved. These may include unknown metabolic factors, changes in neuromuscular function, or in related neurotransmitter systems. Dopaminergic transmission is most likely influenced by activity in the endogenous opioid system and the GABA system. Greater knowledge of the interaction of these and other neuromodulators of less certain significance (e.g., the peptidergic pathways) should provide a better understanding of the pathophysiologic disturbances underlying NMS. Changes in neurotransmission or in skeletal muscle function at the postsynaptic molecular level involving calcium, cyclic adenosine monophosphate, and other intracellular "messengers" also merit investigation and may relate to a final common pathway for heat production in NMS, as discussed in Chapters 3 and 4.

Therapy

The development of elevated body temperature in a patient treated with neuroleptics should always be a cause for concern and prompt medical attention. Apart from NMS, elevated temperatures associated with neuroleptic treatment may result from agranulocytosis, environmentally determined heatstroke, cholestatic jaundice, or other allergic phenomena (Chapter 2). While coincidental febrile illnesses may certainly afflict neuroleptic-treated patients, it is incumbent on the clinician to recognize the potential causal influence of neuroleptic drugs.

When hyperthermia is accompanied by rigidity, deterioration in neurologic status, and autonomic instability, NMS must be considered. Although some authors have recommended postponing consideration of NMS until advanced stages have developed and have based treatment on the relative elevation in temperature, the available clinical data are not precise enough to justify such distinctions reliably. Furthermore, the rapidity of development of NMS in many cases suggests that unnecessary delays in diagnostic evaluation and treatment may be unwise. Thus we recommend that hyperthermia in combination with neurologic changes obliges the clinician to consider stopping neuroleptic drugs until a specific etiology is discovered or until symptoms resolve.

Discontinuation of neuroleptics is significantly correlated with recovery from NMS (Addonizio et al. 1987). In 65 recently reported cases involving oral neuroleptics (and not treated with dantrolene or dopaminergic agonists), the mean ± SD recovery time after drug discontinuation was 9.6 ± 9.1 days (Caroff and Mann 1988); 23 percent recovered in 48 hours, 63 percent by 1 week, 82 percent by 2 weeks, and 97 percent by the end of a month.

Lithium, antidepressants, and medications with potent anticholinergic activity should be discontinued. Whether these drugs offer some prophylactic advantage or, on the contrary, predispose to or complicate NMS is unclear. It may be hazardous to continue lithium in a dehydrated, hyperthermic patient. Similarly, drugs with potent anticholinergic properties may inhibit sweating and further impair heat loss. However, dopamine agonist medication (e.g., amantadine, levodopa) should not be discontinued. Abrupt withdrawal of dopamine agonists may precipitate or exacerbate symptoms in NMS (Simpson and Davis 1984). Their continued use during an acute episode of NMS may, theoretically, decrease the severity of symptoms.

Supportive care should be instituted to reduce hyperthermia (e.g., with antipyretics and a cooling blanket), ensure adequate oxygenation, stabilize the blood pressure, and correct fluid and electrolyte imbalance. The potential severity of dehydration due to sweating and hyperthermia deserves important consideration. Known complications such as thromboembolism, aspiration pneumonia, and cardiorespiratory and renal failure may require special attention, as already mentioned. Tube feedings or administration of medication via nasogastric tube may be necessary in obtunded patients with impaired deglutition. Bedridden and immobile patients may be candidates for antiembolism stockings and minidose heparin therapy to prevent thromboembolism (Lavie et al. 1986a). Simultaneously, an investigation into neurologic, toxic, metabolic, and infectious illnesses should be conducted.

Once NMS is suspected, treatment should be carried out in consultation with an internist or critical care specialist. That treatment be provided by a multidisciplinary team seems crucial. Intensive care monitoring may promote recovery, especially if the patient's medical status is unstable (Janati and Webb 1986). If use of dantrolene is contemplated (see below), consultation with a pharmacist or anesthesiologist may also be helpful. The psychiatrist may play a pivotal role in the early recognition of NMS and prevent premature referral of a "catatonic" patient for psychiatric disposition. In one case of NMS that was initially mistaken for a psychogenic condition, the correct diagnosis was made only after astute intensive care unit staff observed that the patient appeared physically (not mentally) ill (Weinberger and Kelly 1977, oral communication 1985).

Keltner and McIntyre (1985) pointed out several pitfalls and potentially inappropriate nursing actions in the management of patients with NMS. For example, profuse sweating and temperature elevation may be mistaken for flu-like symptoms and lead to treatment with unnecessary medication or medication with anticholinergic properties. Stiffness, catatonic posturing, and akathisia may be mistaken for worsening psychosis and lead to the inappropriate application of restraints, seclusion, and treatment with antipsychotic drugs. Other behaviors may be taken as a sign of denial, manipulation, or malingering, leading staff to ignore or confront the patient.

Special nursing measures are required when the patient becomes ataxic or immobile; requires intubation, dialysis, or cardiac monitoring; or becomes dysphagic and requires mouth care, individualized feedings, or nasogastric tube maintenance (Weiden and Harrigan 1986). The combination of rigidity, akinesia, incontinence, and diaphoresis makes patients with NMS a high risk for developing skin breakdown. Careful skin care, physiotherapy as tolerated, and frequent position changes may lessen the risk of skin and muscle necrosis (Cahill and Arana 1986). Patience and psychiatric expertise are imperative in dealing with patients who have NMS because they are frequently mute and may be delirious, agitated, or psychotic. In view of the need to avoid neuroleptics, agitated or disruptive behaviors should be controlled with benzodiazepine sedatives.

Beyond discontinuing the offending neuroleptic, treating symptoms, and pursuing an investigation into organic illnesses, there is no consensus or rationale as to what measures, if any, should be taken next. Since NMS may not respond well to conventional therapy, the use of specific drugs to facilitate recovery has received increasing attention (Lazarus 1986a) (Table 1.13). Efforts have focused on restoring neurotransmission with a centrally acting agent and on alleviating muscular rigidity with a direct-acting drug. Although not uniformly successful, four drugs (dantrolene and the dopamine agonists amantadine, bromocriptine, and carbidopa/levodopa) have emerged to merit special consideration in the therapy of NMS.

Although these drugs appear promising, it is difficult to evaluate their relative efficacy in comparison to supportive treatment alone because of the lack of control patients in clinical reports, incomplete reporting of data, and variations in route, dosage, and timing of drug administration. More systematic data on drug efficacy could be obtained only from a multicenter collaborative study. However, while this may provide a sufficient sample of patients, ethical problems may complicate the design of a randomized, controlled trial of drug treatment in NMS. For example, is it ethical to withhold dantrolene or bromocriptine, which have been effective in case reports, in treating a patient with a potentially life-threatening episode of NMS?

TABLE 1.13. Specific Drug Therapy of NMS

Drug	Dose/24 hour (mg)[a]	Response			Recovery Time (Days)[a]	
		+	−	±	Total NMS	After Drug
Supportive treatment	—	—	—	—	10 ± 9	—
Bromocriptine	21 ± 12	33	0	4	13 ± 11	3 ± 4
Dantrolene	240 ± 145	33	6	4	8 ± 8	2 ± 2
Levodopa	388 ± 141	8	3	0	31 ± 20	3 ± 1
Amantadine	223 ± 44	8	5	3	14 ± 13	—

[a] Mean ± SD.

Dantrolene

Dantrolene, a long-acting antispasticity drug, has had widespread application in NMS, having been reported to be effective in 33 cases (Caroff and Mann 1988). The drug, a hydantoin derivative, may affect the release of calcium ions from muscle sarcoplasmic reticulum, thus inhibiting the excitation-contraction coupling process and producing relaxation (Ward et al. 1986). By affecting the contractile response of muscle, dantrolene may reduce the hyperthermia in NMS generated by skeletal muscle rigidity.

Hyperthermic hypercatabolic conditions similar to NMS, as seen in malignant hyperthermia (Kolb et al. 1982), heatstroke (Lydiatt and Hill 1981), and toxic reactions from L-asparaginase (Smithson et al. 1983) and phenelzine (Kaplan et al. 1986; Verrilli et al. 1987) have also responded to dantrolene. Not all patients with NMS have benefited from dantrolene (Blue et al. 1986; Downey et al. 1984; Kimsey et al. 1983), however, and in one case (Coons et al. 1982) improvement may have been coincidental. Moreover, dantrolene does not appear to inhibit fluphenazine-induced muscle contractions in vitro (Caroff et al. 1983), although clinical relevance of these in vitro effects has not been established. Ineffectiveness of dantrolene might be related to high temperature and depletion of intracellular adenosine triphosphate from prolonged rigidity, which result in maintenance of contraction independent of calcium concentration (Fuchs 1975). Similarly, fluphenazine-induced contraction might involve simultaneous inhibition of calcium-calmodulin function (Weiss et al. 1982).

Although dantrolene appears to have no appreciable central action, sedation, headache, and other central effects may occur. Furthermore, Patti and colleagues (1981) found that dantrolene increased GABA production in the CNS of rats. Thus potentiation of GABA in the striatum by dantrolene may be partly responsible for its efficacy in NMS (Fricchione 1985).

Patients who respond to dantrolene usually do so rapidly. Normalization of temperature and oxygen consumption may be seen within 48 hours, along with a decline in CPK levels (May et al. 1983). In some instances, defervescence within 1 or 2 hours has been observed (Goekoop and Carbaat 1982). This is encouraging since, as in heatstroke, lethal complications in NMS may be related to the severity and duration of hyperthermia.

Dantrolene may be administered orally or intravenously, the latter route being preferred in uncooperative patients or to quickly counteract thermogenesis. Because of the limited number of reports, the optimal dosage of dantrolene in NMS has not yet been established. In the treatment of malignant hyperthermia, initial intravenous dosages of 1 to 2 mg/kg are recommended, and as much as 10 mg/kg may be required (Kolb et al. 1982; Nelson and Flewellen 1983). In NMS, similar dosage regimens have proved effective, ranging from single intravenous bolus doses of 1 to 10 mg/kg, and divided oral doses ranging from 50 to 600 mg/day.

Varia and Taska (1984) recommended an oral dose of dantrolene of 100 mg four times daily for 1 to 5 days. When oral administration is not possible, Mueller (1985) recommended intravenous administration of dantrolene at dosages of 0.25 to 3 mg/kg qid. Bismuth et al. (1984) felt that dosages below 2 mg/kg were probably ineffective and suggested dosages ranging from 4 to 10 mg/kg qid. Because hepatotoxicity may occur with therapeutic doses (Goulon et al. 1983; Konikoff et al. 1984) or with long-term use (Utili et al. 1977), liver function tests should be monitored closely, and the drug should be discontinued if significant toxicity develops. However, to date there have been no instances of severe or irreversible hepatotoxicity in patients with NMS treated with dantrolene.

Dopamine Agonists

Three dopamine agonists have proved useful in treating

NMS: amantadine, an indirect dopamine agonist; bromocriptine, a direct dopamine agonist; and carbidopa/levodopa, a dopamine precursor. Attempts to treat NMS with dopamine agonists that will reverse the dopamine receptor blockade associated with NMS derive not only from theoretical considerations but also from experience in the treatment of other dopamine deficiency states, such as those underlying Parkinson's disease and dystonia (Lang 1985). In addition, treatment with dopamine agonists appeared to be beneficial in one patient with akinetic mutism due to damage in hypothalamic dopaminergic pathways (Ross and Stewart 1981).

Amantadine has been effective in eight reported NMS cases and ineffective in five (Caroff and Mann 1988). It is typically given in oral doses of 100 mg, two or three times daily. Amantadine has known efficacy in the treatment of catatonic reactions (without fever) secondary to neuroleptics and seems to be superior to anticholinergics in this regard (Gelenberg and Mandel 1977). Anticholinergic and central side effects of amantadine are generally mild (Borison 1983). Furthermore, unlike bromocriptine and carbidopa/levodopa, amantadine rarely worsens the psychosis of schizophrenic patients (Nestelbaum et al. 1986). This is probably due to the relatively selective action of amantadine in the basal ganglia, with fewer dopaminergic effects on mesolimbic and mesocortical structures (Allen 1983).

On the other hand, treatment with bromocriptine and carbidopa/levodopa may be more effective than amantadine because these drugs have a more direct agonist effect on nigrostriatal dopamine receptors. Many cases in which bromocriptine has been effective indicate that it has an onset of action within hours (Dhib-Jalbut et al. 1987; Janati and Webb 1986). A therapeutic response to bromocriptine has been achieved with total daily dosages in the range of 7.5 to 45 mg, usually given in three divided doses. Bromocriptine was effective in 33 cases of NMS, and partially or equivocally effective in an additional four cases (Caroff and Mann 1988).

In one study (Janati and Webb 1986), four patients responded within 24 to 48 hours of therapy, evidenced by rapid defervescence and decreased CPK levels, improved conversational speech, and resolution of extrapyramidal and autonomic symptoms. Bromocriptine is probably the treatment of choice in treating pregnant women who develop NMS (James 1988).

Regardless of which dopamine agonist is used, once symptoms respond, therapy should probably be maintained for at least 10 days and then withdrawn gradually over a week (Hamburg et al. 1986; Mueller 1985). During this time, patients should be monitored carefully for return of symptoms, especially in those patients who developed NMS while receiving long-acting depot neuroleptic preparations or dopamine-depleting agents. Although in some cases it has been argued that improvement with dopamine agonists has been coincidental, compared with the natural course of NMS, the evidence suggests a therapeutic role for these drugs, especially bromocriptine, in the management of NMS. However, based on clinical reports for all drugs, it is difficult to demonstrate significant changes in the overall duration of NMS episodes (Table 1.13) in view of the lack of controls in these reports.

Combination Dantrolene and Dopamine Agonists

The combination of dantrolene and bromocriptine has proven valuable in two cases, possibly due to a complementary effect that is obtained when the two drugs are used together. Through its peripheral effect, dantrolene counteracts the source of hyperthermia in muscle; bromocriptine may reduce hyperthermia through central pathways by restoring dopaminergic transmission in the striatum, hence alleviating rigidity and heat production associated with rigidity, and by exerting direct actions on heat dissipation through thermoregulatory centers in the hypothalamus (Cox 1979). Both

Granato and associates (1983) and Rosse and Ciolino (1985) reported favorable outcomes with this combination of drugs. Because of the potentially more serious adverse reactions due to dantrolene, Mueller (1985) recommended reserving dantrolene for short-term intravenous use in dysphagic patients and then discontinuing it when oral bromocriptine could be given, although both drugs may be given via nasogastric tube. Other authors have recommended a graded approach to therapy in NMS. Lazarus (1986a) recommended dantrolene in cases of NMS complicated by severe hyperthermia, and dopamine agonists in cases manifesting severe extrapyramidal rigidity. In cases manifesting both marked hyperthermia and rigidity, Lazarus (1986a) suggested therapy with dantrolene in combination with a dopaminergic agent. Similarly, Fogel and Goldberg (1985) recommended amantadine and benzodiazepines for mild extrapyramidal symptoms such as rigidity, and confusion without CPK elevation or hyperthermia; dantrolene, bromocriptine, or the combination were recommended when confusion and rigidity were accompanied by hyperthermia, increased CPK, myoglobinuria, or markedly abnormal vital signs. Levinson and Simpson (1986) recommended adding dantrolene when response to dopamine agonists does not occur promptly in patients with fever, obtundation, and hypertension unresponsive to anticholinergics.

Electroconvulsive Therapy

Observations regarding ECT in NMS are limited in scope compared to the number of cases in which pharmacotherapy was employed. Mixed results have been reported with ECT, ranging from clinical improvement to questionable efficacy to lack of efficacy and coma (Addonizio and Susman 1987). Cardiac arrest has occurred in two cases (Hughes 1986; Regestein et al. 1977), and self-limiting atrial arrhythmias developed in two others (Lazarus 1986b; Ries and Schuckit 1980).

In those cases where ECT was effective, the therapeutic effects often emerged immediately, particularly defervescence and decreased rigidity (Jessee and Anderson 1983; Lazarus 1986b; Casey 1988). The rationale for using ECT in NMS may be related to its effectiveness in reversing catatonic reactions (see Chapter 5) and on its ability to increase responsiveness of dopamine receptors in the brain to available dopamine (Modigh et al. 1986). Also, ECT has alleviated rigidity in depressed parkinsonian patients, independent of its antidepressant effect (Asnis 1977; Lebensohn and Jenkins 1975). Sackeim and colleagues (1983) postulated that GABA transmission is enhanced with ECT; thus the efficacy of ECT in NMS may be moderated through the dopamine/GABA interaction (Fricchione 1985).

Patients with NMS who are given ECT should have their cardiac status closely monitored. Neuroleptics (e.g., droperidol) used in anesthesia should be avoided. Succinylcholine, a depolarizing muscle relaxant frequently used during ECT induction, and a known triggering agent of malignant hyperthermia, can probably be used safely when contemplating ECT for patients with NMS (Addonizio and Susman 1987), although there are concerns about its use (George and Woods 1987). With one exception (Grigg 1988), patients with NMS have undergone general anesthesia without difficulty (Downey et al. 1984; Lotstra et al. 1983). Of course, pretreatment with dantrolene and avoidance of succinylcholine is necessary before giving ECT to a patient with known susceptibility to malignant hyperthermia (Franks et al. 1982; Yacoub and Morrow 1986). This procedure has been followed in NMS as well (Bond 1984; Schulte-Sasse et al. 1985).

George and Woods (1987) reported cardiac arrest due to hyperkalemia following administration of succinylcholine in a patient with NMS due to haloperidol. In view of continuing controversy over use of succinylcholine in patients with NMS, cardiac problems, and legal restrictions associated with ECT, ECT appears less promising than pharmacotherapy in the treatment of NMS. However, ECT may be of value in patients with NMS who fail supportive or drug treatment.

Also, in some cases, ECT has been used as a treatment option for patients who continue to be psychotic after resolution of NMS (Aizenberg et al. 1985; Greenberg and Gujavarty 1985; Lavie et al. 1986b; Lotstra et al. 1983; Devanand et al. 1988). In such cases, reinstitution of neuroleptics may pose too great a risk of having NMS recur. In one patient with recurrent manic episodes who was refractory to treatment with lithium and at risk for NMS when exposed to neuroleptics, ECT helped relieve both the mania and symptoms of NMS (Frances and Susman 1986).

Finally, Addonizio and Susman (1987) recommended ECT as an alternative for the patient who presents a "catatonic dilemma." The difficulty in such cases is determining whether neuroleptic-treated patients who develop fever, rigidity, confusion, and autonomic dysfunction actually have NMS or have a catatonic syndrome unrelated to the use of neuroleptics (e.g., catatonic schizophrenia or lethal catatonia). Increased neuroleptic dosage would aggravate NMS but might improve some cases of functional catatonia, although advanced stages of lethal catatonia are probably refractory to treatment with neuroleptics (Mann et al. 1986). On the other hand, withholding neuroleptics would result in improvement in NMS but possible continued deterioration in the catatonic state. When this serious dilemma arises it is essential to stop neuroleptic drugs and consider pharmacologic treatment for NMS. If there is no improvement, then ECT should be considered based on the reasoning that persisting clinical signs may represent underlying functional catatonia that may respond preferentially to ECT (see Chapter 5).

Other Treatments

The use of benzodiazepines in NMS has been advocated based on their efficacy in a small number of patients

(Fricchione et al. 1983; Lew and Tollefson 1983). In many patients with NMS, however, benzodiazepines have had only transient disinhibiting effects and no substantive effect on the course of the syndrome. Yet treatment with benzodiazepines has been effective for patients suffering from functional catatonia, including mutism (Heuser and Benkert 1986; McEvoy and Lohr 1984; Salam et al. 1987), suggesting that some aspects of the NMS symptom complex may be responsive to these agents. Benzodiazepines are remarkably safe, even when used in high doses (Nestoros et al. 1983). In addition to possibly ameliorating symptoms of NMS, benzodiazepines might help modify and control psychotic or agitated behavior (Arana et al. 1986).

Curare (Morris et al. 1980) and the nondepolarizing curariform neuromuscular-blocking agents pancuronium (Sangal and Dimitrijevic 1985) and atracurium (Patel and Bristow 1987) have been used in NMS to control muscle rigidity. In the case reported by Morris et al. (1980), the patient died due to septic complications, whereas in the cases reported by Sangal and Dimitrijevic (1985) and Patel and Bristow (1987), the patients eventually recovered. Because of the muscle-paralyzing properties of these drugs, patients will require adequate sedation and tracheal intubation with positive pressure ventilation (Sieber and McShane 1985).

The combination of intravenous sodium nitroprusside (3 to 4 mcg/kg/min) and oral minoxidil (10 mg every 8 hours) was used to lower blood pressure and temperature in an NMS patient after dantrolene had failed (Blue et al. 1986). These potent antihypertensive agents apparently lowered the patient's temperature by increasing cutaneous heat loss through vasodilation. Blue et al. (1986) felt that nitroprusside would be effective in NMS when peripheral vasoconstriction rather than muscle rigidity predominated.

Nesemann et al. (1984) reported a patient with NMS in whom nitroprusside had no effect on blood pressure or temperature. However, therapy with verapamil, a calcium channel blocker, led to rapid defervescence and the beginning of overall improvement. Pearlman (1986) speculated on a role for calcium channel-blocking agents in NMS based on their ability to reduce levels of intracellular calcium and possibly by displacing neuroleptics from dopamine receptors, as reported by DeVries and Beart (1985).

Lastly, there was one case of NMS that was successfully treated with pridinolum mesylate, a peripheral anticholinergic muscle relaxant (Giordani et al. 1985). Another patient showed marked improvement with benztropine after pretreatment with bromocriptine (Schvehla and Herjanic (1988). In general, however, anticholinergics, antihistamines, and amobarbital have been ineffective in NMS. Furthermore, because anticholinergics inhibit sweating and impair heat dissipation, they may contribute to hyperthermia in NMS.

By discontinuing the offending neuroleptic and providing supportive therapy, symptoms in NMS usually remit within 1 to 2 weeks (Table 1.13). The syndrome may last longer if depot neuroleptics are responsible. Remission of symptoms does not guarantee complete recovery. Patients have relapsed following premature discontinuation of therapy (Hamburg et al. 1986; Janati and Webb 1986).

The treatment of NMS may be complicated by the reemergence of psychosis when neuroleptics are discontinued. Several authors have addressed this problem (Aizenberg et al. 1985; Pelonero et al. 1985; Shalev and Munitz 1986; Levenson and Fisher 1988; Susman and Addonizio 1988). First, it is necessary to ask whether no treatment or treatment other than neuroleptics will suffice, for example, lithium, carbamazepine, benzodiazepines, or ECT. This would be based on a careful diagnostic reassessment of the case. If not, then the available data indicate choosing a neuroleptic from a different chemical class than the one that caused NMS, preferably a low-potency neuroleptic, such as thioridazine. Only one (10 percent) of 10 patients had recurrent NMS when rechallenged with thioridazine, whereas six (75 percent) of eight patients had recurrent episodes when rechallenged with the same drug, according to a review by Shalev and Munitz

(1986). Moreover, rechallenge with other neuroleptics of the same potency as the drug that originally precipitated NMS resulted in recurrence of NMS in five (83 percent) of six patients, with two fatalities (Shalev and Munitz 1986).

In our review of the literature, among 52 reported NMS patients with a history of previous neuroleptic treatment, 9 (17 percent) had, in retrospect, developed NMS previously (Caroff and Mann 1988). Furthermore, three (21 percent) of 14 patients challenged with the same drug developed a recurrence of NMS. Regardless of the initial triggering agent, 10 (48 percent) of 21 patients developed a second episode of NMS when challenged with a high-potency drug, whereas NMS recurred in only four (15 percent) of 26 patients who were challenged with a low-potency neuroleptic. Overall, among 47 reported cases in which neuroleptic treatment was reinstituted, 14 (30 percent) developed recurrent episodes. These data support the triggering role of neuroleptics, although other factors appear to be operative in determining the development of NMS at a particular time. Moreover, recurrences appear to correlate more closely with the dopamine antagonist potency of the drug involved.

When restarting a neuroleptic, a candid discussion should be held and documented with the patient and the patient's family to inform them of risks and alternatives. Prophylactic use of oral dantrolene or bromocriptine during rechallenge has been suggested (White 1984), and dantrolene has been reported as possibly successful in one case (Lesser et al. 1986). It is prudent to avoid "prn" (as needed) administration of neuroleptics, since such treatment may contribute to the development of NMS (Campbell and Simpson 1986). The use of an aggressive loading schedule should also be avoided (Shalev and Munitz 1986). Potent neuroleptics should be used cautiously in psychotic patients with underlying mood disorders. All patients should be kept well hydrated and have their vital signs and physical condition monitored carefully in the hospital for development of fever, tachycardia, diaphoresis, confusion, muscular rigidity, and CPK elevation. Neuroleptics should be stopped at the first sign of recurrence of NMS, and one of the alternative treatments above should be considered. Therapeutic guidelines in NMS may change as experience accumulates and the pathophysiology of this disorder becomes more completely understood.

Conclusion

NMS is one of the most serious adverse reactions to neuroleptic drug treatment. This underrecognized and incompletely understood complication of neuroleptic therapy is rare but may be life threatening. Core features of NMS consist of rigidity, hyperthermia, autonomic disturbances, and impaired mental status, although there is considerable heterogeneity of clinical symptoms. NMS is not simply misdiagnosed lethal catatonia, nor can it be explained in the majority of cases as resulting from infections or other medical conditions. There are no pathognomonic laboratory or autopsy findings. The syndrome appears to be mediated by dopamine receptor blockade at various levels in the CNS; however, neurotransmitters other than dopamine may be involved. In addition, neuroleptic-induced alterations in skeletal muscle function may contribute to the development of NMS. NMS may represent the neuroleptic-induced subtype of a more generalized and non-specific *syndrome malin*, which may be provoked by other psychotropic agents and a variety of medical disorders.

Along with prompt cessation of neuroleptics and symptomatic treatment, the combination of dantrolene and postsynaptic dopamine agonists currently appears to be the most effective therapy in NMS. An apparent decline in mortality since 1980 may reflect earlier diagnosis and more specific treatment. However, it is difficult to assess the various treatments due to limitations inherent in evaluting data from single case reports and to the tendency to report only positive results. There are no controlled outcome studies in NMS, and their implementation may raise serious methodological and ethical concerns. Furthermore, there is a significant risk of recurrence on rechallenge with neuroleptics. Additional studies are needed to develop an animal model of NMS. The investigation of low-dose neuroleptic regimens, alternatives to neuroleptic therapy, and reliable early predictive signs of NMS is also important. Although considerable progress has been made in understanding NMS based on clinical experience, there remains a compelling need for additional basic science and clinical investigations in NMS to elucidate pathophysiologic mechanisms and to devise more effective therapeutic strategies.

Chapter 2

Neuroleptic-Related Heatstroke

Chapter 2

Neuroleptic-Related Heatstroke

*T*wo hyperthermic syndromes besides neuroleptic malignant syndrome (NMS) have been described in association with neuroleptic treatment: so-called benign hyperthermia and neuroleptic-related heatstroke (NRHS). Benign hyperthermia has been viewed as an immunological-mediated drug fever (Kick 1981) or, alternatively, as the product of mild neuroleptic-induced thermoregulatory impairment (Belfer and Shader 1970). It occurs during the first 2 weeks of treatment, is usually associated with mild non-life-threatening temperature elevation, and is brief in duration. Benign hyperthermia has been reported to develop in 0.7 to 5.7 percent of patients starting neuroleptic treatment, although 10 to 15 percent of patients beginning clozapine appear to be affected (Davis 1985; Kick 1981).

In contrast, NRHS and NMS represent potentially lethal complications of neuroleptic treatment. Both disorders appear underrecognized, share a number of clinical features, and may be confused with a host of other hyperthermic illnesses, including fulminating hyperthermic syndromes related to therapy with psychotropic agents other than neuroleptics (see Chapter 3). Furthermore, NRHS and NMS resemble clinical descriptions of non-drug-related lethal catatonia (Chapter 5).

In this chapter, the physiology of normal thermoregulation will be reviewed, and recent data indicating a prominent role for dopamine in central thermoregulation will be presented. These data suggest that neuroleptics can promote hyperthermia by blocking dopamine-mediated central thermoregulatory heat-loss pathways in hot environments or during excessive endogenous heat production. The concept of "fever" as a discrete subtype of hyperthermia differing physiologically from other types of temperature elevation due to pathologic or pharmacologic impairment of thermoregulatory mechanisms will be emphasized. The clinical presentation of heatstroke will be described, and the social, behavioral, and medical factors that place psychiatric patients at increased risk for heatstroke will be reviewed. In addition to the role of neuroleptic effects on central dopaminergic heat-loss pathways in the etiology of NRHS, the contribution of peripheral anticholinergic activity of neuroleptics themselves, or of anticholinergic drugs administered concurrently, will be explored.

Normal Thermoregulation

Warm-blooded animals are generally able to maintain body temperature within narrow limits despite large variations in ambient temperature (Brück 1983; Guyton 1986). This is accomplished by a highly effective homeostatic control system in which cutaneous and core thermosensors monitor the body's thermal state and transmit this information to a central controller (Figure 2.1). Here, converging central and peripheral temperature signals are integrated and compared with the "set point." The set point represents an optimal steady-state temperature at which no thermoregulatory responses are activated. If the controller detects a change in body temperature away from the set point, it activates autonomic and behavioral thermoregulatory effectors to counteract that change. The set point is generally conceptualized as an endogenous reference signal generated independent of core body temperature by neurons located within the central nervous system (CNS) interface between thermosensors and thermoeffectors.

The anterior hypothalamic preoptic area (AH/POA) represents the most important component in the central thermoregulatory control system and is the first structure to detect and respond to a departure of body temperature away from the set point (Satinoff 1978). Although other CNS thermoregulatory sites throughout the brain stem and spinal cord are capable of integrating local thermal information with information from peripheral thermoreceptors (Boulant 1980), the AH/POA serves to coordinate and adjust the activity of these lower centers. Without its input, thermoregulatory responses at the most caudal sites would be activated only at extremely hot or cold temperatures. Many AH/POA neurons are locally thermosensitive. In addition, the AH/POA receives input from thermosensors in the skin, brain stem, spinal cord, and deep body viscera.

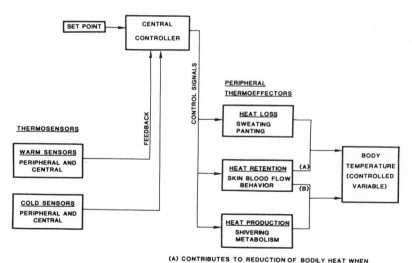

(A) CONTRIBUTES TO REDUCTION OF BODILY HEAT WHEN EITHER CENTRAL OR PERIPHERAL TEMPERATURE RISES ABOVE THE THERMONEUTRAL ZONE.

(B) CONTRIBUTES TO INCREASE OF BODILY HEAT WHEN EITHER CENTRAL OR PERIPHERAL TEMPERATURE FALLS BELOW THE THERMONEUTRAL ZONE.

FIGURE 2.1. Block diagram of thermoregulation. Adapted from Brück (1983), with permission.

Warm-sensitive neurons located within the AH/POA may be divided into three groups based on their ranges of firing rates at 38 °C: low-firing, medium-firing, and high-firing neurons (Boulant 1980). The lowest-firing group have the greatest thermosensitivity in the hyperthermic range. Cold sensitive neurons within the AH/POA are locally thermosensitive and, in addition increase their firing rate both in response to input from cutaneous and spinal cold receptors, and reduced inhibition by AH/POA warm receptors in the cold (Scott and Boulant 1984).

Figure 2.2 provides a neuronal model of how AH/POA neurons may integrate central and peripheral thermal signals activating effector mechanisms for heat loss and heat gain. Since low-firing warm sensitive AH/POA neurons are

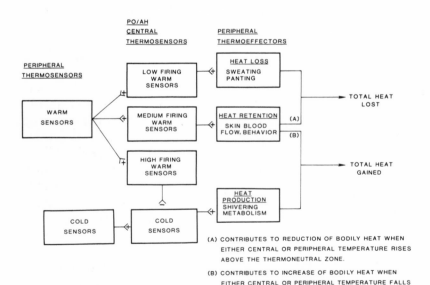

FIGURE 2.2. Neuronal model of thermoregulation. Adapted from Boulant (1980), with permission.

sensitive only at hot AH/POA temperatures, they, along with peripheral warm receptors, control heat loss mechanisms operative in the heat: panting and, particularly in humans, sweating. Similarly, high-firing warm sensitive AH/POA neurons, which are not sensitive to AH/POA warming but decrease their firing rates with AH/POA cooling, leading to reduced inhibition of cold receptors, are, along with peripheral cold receptors, involved in heat production mechanisms in the cold: nonshivering thermogenesis, and, in humans, primarily shivering thermogenesis.

Heat retention responses relate to those thermoeffector mechanisms that are most active in the thermoneutral range and that are the first to respond when body temperature is altered above or below the set point. Skin blood flow is the principal autonomic thermoeffector mechanism involved in heat retention. Control of skin blood flow is mediated by medium-firing warm sensitive AH/POA neurons, whose activity is maximal in the thermoneutral range.

In addition to autonomic mechanisms, heat retention is maintained by behavioral thermoregulation, which is particularly important near thermoneutrality. The AH/POA has both afferent and efferent connections with various limbic areas and pathways that participate in the emotional coloring of sensory input. These limbic components evaluate integrated information from central and peripheral thermoreceptors as "thermally" comfortable or uncomfortable and initiate compensatory behavioral responses. Recently, the hippocampus has been implicated as selectively exciting these same medium-firing warm sensitive AH/POA neurons with maximal activity at thermoneutrality (Boulant and Demieville 1977).

Unlike the AH/POA, the posterior hypothalamus appears to contain a minimal number of locally thermosensitive neurons. Although it receives input from skin and spinal thermosensors, its role as an integrator of thermosensory input is probably limited (Myers 1980). Rather, it receives incoming signals for thermoeffector responses from the

AH/POA and extrahypothalamic structures, and activates thermoeffectors for heat loss, heat retention, and heat production.

In humans, sweating and increased skin blood flow, along with behavioral modifications, are the thermoeffector mechanisms active at high ambient temperatures. Three major avenues are available for dissipation of bodily heat: radiation of heat through space, convection and conduction to air currents, and evaporation of sweat. Heat loss to air currents reaches a maximum as wind velocity approaches 15 to 20 miles per hour, and evaporation is facilitated by a dry environment. As the ambient temperature approaches that of the body, radiation, convection, and conduction will yield a net heat gain rather than a heat loss, leaving evaporation as the only major mechanism of heat loss. Sweat glands, under the control of sympathetic nerves that have muscarinic endings rather than adrenergic endings, provide water to be vaporized by heat brought to the body surface by dilated peripheral vessels. However, high humidity will impair this mechanism because less sweat can be lost to the already highly saturated air. Thus continuous heat storage may occur in a hot, windless, and humid environment. Since vulnerability to heat storage may be offset by acclimatization, which requires several weeks of exposure to heat to develop, sudden rises in ambient temperature during heat waves can present a particular problem.

Role of Dopamine in Thermoregulation

In 1971 Bligh and associates proposed a model for the involvement of monoamines in mammalian hypothalamic thermoregulation (Figure 2.3). Data were derived through intracerebroventricular (ICV) injections of serotonin, acetylcholine, and norephinephrine in sheep, goats, and rabbits. Two principal pathways between thermoreceptors and thermoregulators were described. One was from warm sensors to heat loss effectors, and the other from cold sensors to heat production effectors. Since heat production is reduced by exposure to heat, and heat loss is reduced by exposure to cold, crossed inhibitory pathways were included between the two main pathways. In this model, serotonin acts along the pathway from warm sensors to heat loss effectors activating heat loss mechanisms of panting and vasodilation, and inhibiting shivering. Acetylcholine acts along the pathway from cold sensors to heat production effectors activating shivering, causing vasoconstriction, and decreasing panting. Norephinephrine functions as an inhibitor between the two main pathways, suppressing all thermoeffector mechanisms active at a given ambient temperature.

Dopamine was not included in the Bligh et al. (1971) model. Pharmacological support for a role for dopamine in central thermoregulation originated from evidence that central and systemic injections of specific dopamine agonists such as apomorphine and amantadine could lower body temperature in rodents maintained at 20 °C or below (Cox and Lee 1977; Cox and Tha 1975; Yehuda and Wurtman 1975). Hypothermia produced in this manner could be blocked by specific dopamine antagonists such as pimozide (Cox and Lee 1977). Similar studies in sheep and goats indicated that ICV injection of dopamine caused hypothermia, which was also blocked by dopamine antagonists (De Roij et al. 1977, 1978a). Moreover, amphetamine, an indirect dopamine agonist, caused a similar hypothermia at low

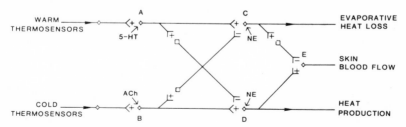

FIGURE 2.3. Role of serotonin (5-HT), norepinephrine (NE), and acetylcholine (ACh) in the control of body temperature in sheep. Adapted from Bligh et al. (1971), with permission.

ambient temperatures (Yehuda and Wurtman 1975). However, in these studies, agents were administered either systemically or intracerebroventricularly, leaving their exact site of action unclear. Also, experiments involving dopamine agonists and antagonists relied heavily on the assumption that these agents were not simply acting on noradrenergic receptors. Furthermore, studies with dopamine agonists failed to demonstrate a role for endogenous dopamine in the central thermoregulatory mediation of heat loss since they had been performed at or below room temperature, where an endogenous heat loss system would probably be inactive.

In experiments involving intrahypothalamic injections of dopamine in the rat (Cox and Lee 1980; Cox et al. 1978) and cat (Ruwe and Myers 1978), the AH/POA site most sensitive for dopamine-mediated hypothermia was precisely identified within the medial preoptic area. The primary innervation of this site appears to be derived from hypothalamic neurons of the rostral incertohypothalamic group located in the periventricular region of the anterior hypothalamus (A14) (Gonzalez et al. 1986; Moore 1987). Furthermore, Cox and Lee (1980) and Ruwe and Myers (1978) were able to identify in the rat and cat, respectively, AH/POA norephinephrine-sensitive hypothermic sites located away from the dopamine-sensitive sites, confirming that dopamine agonists and antagonists do not cause hypothermia through actions on noradrenergic mechanisms.

Cox and associates (1978, 1980) were able to demonstrate a role for endogenous dopamine as a central mediator of heat loss by employing bilateral injections of the dopamine antagonists pimozide and haloperidol into the preoptic area of rats exposed to an infrared lamp-imposed heat load. Under such circumstances, an endogenous heat loss system would be expected to be activated. Prior to dopamine antagonist treatment, rats responded to the imposed heat load by vasodilation of tail skin blood vessels, yielding an increase in tail skin temperature, but little increase in core body temperature. Following dopamine antagonist treatment, rats had a reduced rise in tail temperature on heat exposure and a significant elevation in core body temperature, consistent with a physiologic role for endogenous dopamine in mediating heat loss. Further studies by this group of investigators have indicated that dopamine plays a far more prominent role than norepinephrine in AH/POA heat loss mediation. Recent electrophysiologic studies examining the firing rate and thermosensitivity of individual AH/POA neurons perfused with dopamine have shown that dopamine excites a large portion of warm sensitive neurons and inhibits cold sensivite neurons (Scott and Boulant 1984).

De Roij et al. (1978b) provided evidence for the involvement of serotonin in dopamine receptor-mediated changes in core body temperature. They noted that in goats maintained at an ambient temperature of 20 °C, ICV injection of both dopamine (800 μ g) and serotonin (800 μ g) caused a decreased body temperature and dilation of ear vessels. While the thermoregulatory response at 20 °C to ICV administration of dopamine could be blocked by both the serotonin antagonist methysergide and the dopamine antagonist haloperidol, the thermoregulatory response to ICV administration of serotonin could only be blocked by methysergide but not haloperidol. These findings suggested that dopamine receptor-mediated hypothermia results from dopaminergic stimulation of serotonin release, which, in turn, activates heat loss effectors. Cox and Lee (1979) were able to localize such a dopamine/serotonin link in the rat to the previously identified dopamine-sensitive site for hypothermia within the AH/POA. Similar to findings in the goat, Cox et al. (1980) reported that methysergide in the rat reduced the hypothermic response to central injection of both dopamine and serotonin, whereas haloperidol blocked only the response to dopamine.

The accumulated evidence suggested that dopamine should replace norephinephrine in at least some of the hypothalamic synapses occupied by norepinephrine in the original Bligh et al. (1971) model of mammalian thermoregulation. The findings suggested that a probable location for dopaminergic heat loss pathway would be before the serotonin synapse in the Bligh et al. (1971) model as indicated in Figure 2.4. While the cell bodies of these serotonin-containing neurons are probably located in the midbrain Raphe nuclei, it seems likely that dopamine acts on their nerve terminals in the AH/POA (Cox et al. 1980).

Studies by De Roij and associates (1978b, 1979) have suggested the involvement of two types of dopamine receptors in central thermoregulation: in the goat, an excitatory dopamine receptor, blocked by treatment with haloperidol and located in the hypothalamic heat loss pathway before the serotonin synapse; and an inhibitory dopamine receptor, not blocked by haloperidol and causing decreased peripheral vasomotor tone. Both pathways could have a physiologic role in heat loss in the heat.

Yamawaki and associates (1983, 1985) have also proposed the existence of two separate dopamine-related thermoregulatory mechanisms, one involving both dopamine and serotonin, and the other involving only dopamine. However, these authors suggested that activation of the dopamine/serotonin thermoregulatory pathway causes hyperthermia rather than hypothermia as reported by Cox and associates (1980), and that it is insensitive to haloperidol blockade rather than blocked by haloperidol as reported by

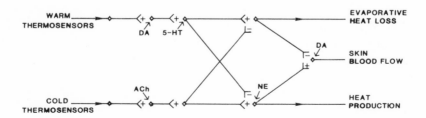

FIGURE 2.4. Incorporation of dopamine (DA) in the neuronal model of thermoregulation. Adapted from De Roij et al. (1978b), with permission.

De Roij and associates (1978b, 1979). These disparities may, in part, be attributable to methodologic difficulties, including nonspecific routes for administering exogenous probes, and selection of an ambient temperature (23 °C) above the 4 to 20 °C at which similar studies were conducted. Still, this raises the intriguing possibility of a neuroleptic-insensitive dopamine/serotonin hyperthermic pathway that could be blocked by serotonin antagonists but enhanced by neuroleptic blockade of the haloperidol-sensitive dopaminergic heat loss mechanism, as discussed in Chapter 3.

Along with the AH/POA, the nigrostriatal dopamine system may be involved in dopamine-mediated heat loss mechanisms (Lee et al. 1985). Bilateral apomorphine injections into the substantia nigra of the rat produced a dose-related hypothermia that was almost identical in magnitude and time course to the same dosage of apomorphine injected bilaterally into the AH/POA (Brown et al. 1982). Hypothermia was blocked by bilateral injections of pimozide into the substantia nigra. Furthermore, bilateral electrolytic lesioning of the substantia nigra has been associated with significant hyperthermia in rats exposed to heat (Brown et al. 1982).

Thus the substantia nigra might represent a "lower" thermoregulatory center (Satinoff 1978) caudal to the AH/POA, as discussed earlier. Consistent with this schema, the substantia nigra would be expected to transmit thermoregulatory impulses to the more rostral AH/POA, in addition to its local role in thermoregulation. In support of this, Kiyohara et al. (1984) have demonstrated a direct projection from the substantia nigra to the AH/POA, and some hypothalamic dopaminergic neurons have been shown to have their cell bodies in the substantia nigra (Javoy-Agid et al. 1984). Alternatively, the major thermoregulatory role of the substantia nigra may involve activation of heat loss mechanisms in response to impulses from the AH/POA (Lee et al. 1985) transmitted through a pathway from the AH/POA to the substantia nigra as described by Swanson (1976). Lee and associates (1985) have suggested that transmission from the substantia nigra to the midbrain reticular formation could influence autonomic mechanisms for heat loss, while nigro-striatal projections to the thalamus, and ultimately motor cortex, could facilitate behavioral heat loss.

A consistent finding in studies of mammalian thermoregulation has been that neuroleptics promote poikilothermia, that is, they render animals thermally dependent on their environment, leading to hypothermia in the cold and hyperthermia in the heat (Kollias and Bullard 1964). Departures from this pattern cluster around studies defining hot and cold ambient conditions at temperatures close to thermoneutrality. Agents examined include phenothiazines, butyrophenones, diphenylbutyl-piperidines, and thioxanthines (Clark 1979). The preceding review of dopaminergic thermoregulatory mechanisms indicates that at least certain neuroleptics may promote hyperthermia by interfering with hypothalamic heat loss mediated by endogenous dopamine neurotramsmission.

Neuroleptics are a large group of drugs displaying numerous and differing pharmacologic actions, including varying effects on metabolism, central and peripheral cholinergic, and alpha-adrenergic receptors. All, however, exert significant effects on dopamine receptors. Given the consistent finding of neuroleptic-induced hyperthermia in the heat, and the prominent role of endogenous dopamine in hypothalamic mediation of heat loss, it would seem reasonable to propose that neuroleptics promote hyperthermia by blocking central thermoregulatory pathways involving dopamine receptors (Mann and Greenstein 1983).

The relative potency of individual neuroleptics in causing hyperthermia in animals exposed to heat has not been studied as systematically as has the potency of individual neuroleptics in causing hypothermia in the cold (Maickel 1970). However, data comparing (1) haloperidol and thioridazine in blocking apomorphine-induced hyperthermia in rabbits (Roszell and Horita 1975), (2) pimozide-

and chlorpromazine-induced hyperthermia in rats maintained in the heat (Yehuda and Wurtman 1975), and (3) the ability of various neuroleptics to block amphetamine-induced hypothermia in rats (Yehuda 1979; Yehuda and Frommer 1977) all suggest a correlation between a neuroleptic's potency in blocking central dopaminergic receptors, and its milligram per milligram potency in disrupting central thermoregulatory heat loss mechanisms.

Fever, Hyperthermia, and Heatstroke

In considering elevations in body temperature, it is important to note that the term *fever* refers to a discrete subtype of hyperthermia (Stitt 1979). During fever, endogenous pyrogens produced in response to infections, immunologic reactions, mechanical trauma, and other causes of tissue injury act on the hypothalamus to bring about an elevation in the set point, with a consequent increase in body temperature (Dinarello 1985). Febrile hyperthermia is the product of coordinated effector responses requiring intact central thermoregulatory mechanisms. Other features of fever are: (1) response to aspirin-like drugs, which are prostaglandin inhibitors; (2) lack of response to external cooling alone in the absence of aspirin-like agents (the body's tendency to defend the elevation in temperature dictated by the set-point interval); and (3) the uncommon occurrence of fevers in excess of 41.1 °C. As noted earlier, at least some cases of benign hyperthermia represent a drug fever, that is, a fever resulting from an immunologic reaction to the neuroleptic agent.

In contrast to fever, other types of hyperthermia involve either disordered central thermoregulation, impaired peripheral heat loss, excessive thermal challenge, or a combination of these factors (Clark and Lipton 1984). Antipyretics are ineffective in nonfebrile hyperthermia because pyrogens and prostaglandins are not involved. Nonfebrile hyperthermia occurring independent of a hot environment may be the product of various hypermetabolic disorders such as thyrotoxicosis and pheochromocytoma; cerebral lesions affecting central thermoregulatory centers, including tumors, infections, degenerative diseases, and vascular accidents; and withdrawal from ethanol or sedative-hypnotic drugs. In addition, drugs may alter body temperature by acting on any component of the thermoregulatory system: thermosensors and their afferent pathways, thermoeffectors and their efferent pathways, and coordinating neurons within the CNS (Clark 1979).

Heatstroke is a life-threatening disorder requiring emergency medical treatment. Heatstroke is generally divided into two subtypes: classic and exertional (Table 2.1). Classic heatstroke is characterized by body temperature above 40.6 °C (105 °F); profound CNS dysfunction with severe disorientation, delirium, or coma; and anhydrosis (Anderson et al. 1983). Heatstroke typically occurs in epidemic fashion during summer heat waves. Since during a heat wave elevations in environmental temperature and humidity are sustained over several days, active perspiration is continuous prior to its eventual cessation. Thus the majority of cases come to medical attention only after 3 or more days into the heat wave.

Individuals who are most at risk for classic heatstroke are the elderly. Older adults are predisposed on the basis of chronic illnesses, in particular cardiovascular disease, diabetes mellitus, malnutrition, and acute or chronic alcoholism (Knochel 1985). Other risk factors in the general population include infectious illnesses, severe burns, congenital absence of sweat glands, obesity, chronic inactivity, living on higher floors of multistory buildings, and lack of air-conditioning or access to air-conditioned places (Kilbourne et al. 1982; Knochel 1980).

In sharp contrast to the aged and debilitated patients typically involved in classic heatstroke, exertional heatstroke occurs primarily in nonmedicated, young, healthy individuals with normal thermoregulatory capacity. In this instance, heat produced by muscular work in a hot environment exceeds the body's capacity to dissipate it. In the United States the highest incidence of exertional heatstroke is found in marathon runners, football players, and military recruits (Knochel 1985). Overzealous training, requirements for performance that exceeds human capacity, clothing that prevents vaporization of sweat (e.g., plastic sweatsuits or leather football gear), and inadequate hydration and salt supplementation represent risk factors for the development of exertional heatstroke (Knochel 1980, 1985).

TABLE 2.1. Comparison of Classic and Exertional Heatstroke

	Classic	**Exertional**
Age group affected	Older (or infants)	Young
State of health	+ Predisposing illnesses	Good
Epidemic occurrence	Yes	No
Prevailing weather	Heat wave	Variable
Skin	Dry and hot	50% continue to sweat; skin may appear cool
Acid/base disturbance	Respiratory alkalosis	Lactic acidosis
Rhabdomyolysis	Rare; mild creatine phosphokinase elevations; acute renal failure (rare)	Common, with marked creatine phosphokinase elevations, myoglobinuria, hyperuricemia; 30% develop acute renal failure
Disseminated intravascular coagulation	Rare	Common
Electrolyte disturbances	Hypokalemia	Hyperkalemia, or hypokalemia, hypocalcemia, hyperphosphatemia
Irreversible CNS impairment	Elderly patients seem more susceptible	Somewhat less common

Note. Adapted from Anderson et al. (1983), with permission.

Unlike classic heatstroke, about half of patients with exertional heatstroke continue to sweat in the acute phase. Furthermore, the skin may appear cool despite a high core body temperature. These factors may obscure the proper diagnosis and prevent prompt treatment. Although elevated levels of serum creatine phosphokinase (CPK) may be present in classic heatstroke, they rarely exceed 2,000 IU. In exertional heatstroke, massive muscle damage (rhabdomyolysis) is common, with marked CPK elevations and acute myoglobinuric renal failure in 30 percent of patients. Prominent lactic acidosis is often an early finding, but unlike classic heatstroke, this finding does not carry a poor prognosis. Disseminated intravascular coagulation, often severe in exertional heatstroke, is less pronounced in classic heatstroke.

Both forms of heatstroke may result in myocardial infarction and congestive heart failure, pancreatitis, hepatic failure, and adult respiratory distress syndrome. Mental status changes such as coma, stupor, and agitated delirium are common in both forms. CNS manifestations include grand mal seizures, pupillary abnormalities, and hemiplegia acutely, with cerebellar symptoms including ataxia and dysarthria, a not infrequent permanent complication (Lefkowitz et al. 1983).

Maintenance of muscle tone during heatstroke is variable. A number of authors state that skeletal musculature is typically flaccid, with rigidity developing only following initation of therapeutic cooling (Knochel 1985; Petersdorf 1977). Clark and Lipton (1984) stated that rigidity may develop secondary to hyperthermia during the later stages of heatstroke. Shibolet et al. (1976) noted that "profound rigidity with tonic contractions, coarse tremor, dystonic movement, and muscle cramps often alternate with the convulsive state" (p. 292) during heatstroke. However, increased muscle tone is almost never reported in cases of neuroleptic-related heatstroke (Bark 1982a; Clark and Lipton 1984).

A variety of drugs have been associated with the development of heatstroke. Clark and Lipton (1984) stressed the value of dividing drug-related heatstroke into two broad categories: drug-facilitated heatstroke and drug-induced heatstroke. In drug-facilitated heatstroke, direct effects of drugs on the thermoregulatory system impair its capacity to increase heat loss in response to an imposed heat load. Agents exert only a permissive influence that favors heat storage; the development of hyperthermia hinges on exposure to a hot environment or heat production during strenuous exercise. Neuroleptics and anticholinergics represent two categories of drugs that, at therapeutic dosages, are frequently implicated in drug-facilitated heatstroke. Anticholinergics inhibit sweating, whereas neuroleptics interfere with central thermoregulation, although peripheral anticholinergic effects of neuroleptics may further impair heat loss mechanisms.

Agents involved in drug-induced heatstroke increase endogenous heat production and cause hyperthermia independent of environmental conditions. Drugs may act directly on peripheral effector mechanisms for heat production, for example, increased cellular metabolism associated with salicylate intoxication and anesthetic effects on muscle in malignant hyperthermia (see Chapter 4). Drugs may act directly on the CNS to cause heatstroke as in intoxication with amphetamines, anticholinergics, heterocyclic antidepressants, monoamine oxidase inhibitors, xanthine derivatives, lysergic acid diethylamide (LSD), phencyclidine (PCP), and others. Pathophysiologic mechanisms by which drugs acting directly on the CNS may cause heatstroke are considered in detail in Chapter 3. Included are CNS mechanisms for increased psychomotor activity, enhanced muscle tone, constriction of cutaneous vasculature, and direct drug effects on the hypothalamus.

Neuroleptics clearly exert actions on the hypothalamus. Their suppression of central heat loss pathways appears to be involved in the pathogenesis of both NRHS and NMS (Mann and Greenstein 1983). However, in NMS, excess heat appears derived either from direct effects of neuroleptics on muscle or from neuroleptic-induced extrapyramidal muscular rigidity, whereas in NRHS excess heat is derived from a hot environment. Thus the NMS appears to represent a genuine drug-induced heatstroke. In contrast, NRHS is best viewed as drug-facilitated heatstroke in which neuroleptics simply increase vulnerability to a well-described form of environmental heat illness by interfering with heat dissipation.

Psychiatric Aspects of Heatstroke

Risk Factors

The high prevalence in psychiatric patients of many factors that predispose to both classic and exertional heatstroke places this population at increased risk for its development (Bark 1982b; Lazarus 1985a; Mann and Boger 1978; Tacke and Venglainen 1987; Wise 1973). In the wake of deinstitutionalization, increasing numbers of homeless patients have been exposed to high environmental temperature and humidity during heat waves. Such patients often wear multiple layers of clothing, severely compromising evaporative heat loss. Others live in small, crowded, poorly ventilated or unair-conditioned rooms, often on the top floors of multistory buildings. Poor nutrition or delusional beliefs concerning nutrition may lead to inadequate fluid and salt intake necessary for effective evaporative heat loss.

Hospitalized psychiatric patients are also at increased risk for heatstroke. Many psychiatric inpatient units are not yet air-conditioned. Seclusion rooms represent a specific concern, as they are usually small, hot, and lack cross-ventilation. Increased motor activity associated with agitation, struggling against restraints, and psychotic excitement clearly increase the likelihood of exertional heatstroke (Knochel 1980). The more frequent occurrence of agitation and aggressive behavior in males may in part explain Bark's

(1982a) observation tht NRHS affects nine males to every one female, well above the 2:1 male-to-female ratio for the occurrence of heatstroke in the general population.

Other behavioral characteristics of psychiatric patients may contribute to the risk of heatstroke. It is possible that certain schizophrenic patients do not perceive an excessively hot environment as noxious, and thus fail to remove themselves from it (Kane et al. 1971; Williams 1953). Before the neuroleptic era, it was suggested that schizophrenic patients may be defective in their homeostatic thermoregulatory capacity. Finkelman and Stephens (1936) and Gottlieb and Linder (1935) presented data suggesting that, compared to normal individuals, schizophrenics develop relative hypothermia in the cold and hyperthermia in the heat (i.e., poikilothermia). Curiously, neuroleptics appear to exert similar effects on human and animal thermoregulation.

Role of Neuroleptics

In 1956 Ayd reported a case of fatal heatstroke in a 41-year-old chlorpromazine-treated schizophrenic patient exposed to hot weather. Ayd (1956) discussed evidence that chlorpromazine could impair hypothalamic thermoregulatory mechanisms. He postulated that death in this case was the result of chlorpromazine's effects on the hypothalamus "accentuated by the high environmental temperature" (p. 191).

Zelman and Guillan (1970) reported three similar cases occurring during a heat wave, noting a regrettable lack of reference to NRHS in journals, textbooks, and product information summaries. These authors cited the findings of Kollias and Bullard (1964) that phenothiazine-induced depression of hypothalamic regulation renders rats thermally dependent on their environment, leading to hyperthermia in the heat. Additional case reports of NRHS suggested a similar pattern of neuroleptic-induced thermal dependency in humans.

Recently, NRHS has been reported more frequently, particularly in the context of its delimitation from NMS (Caroff 1980). Bark (1982a) reviewed 48 cases of heatstroke in neuroleptic-treated patients. In 43 patients, hyperthermia was attributed to neuroleptic-induced depression of heat loss mechanisms in the heat. The remaining five cases, however, did not involve high environmental temperatures. Instead, hyperthermia was attributed to exercise, hyperactivity, agitation during sedative-hypnotic withdrawal, and agitation combined with impaired heat dissipation during sheet restraint.

Clark and Lipton (1984) reviewed 45 cases of NRHS involving a maximal body temperature of at least 40 °C. Most of these cases had also been reviewed in Bark's (1982a) series. Clark and Lipton (1984) concluded that among drug-related hyperthermias, NRHS most closely mimics classic heatstroke rather than exertional heatstroke in phenomenology and pathophysiology. Of the 45 cases, only six had maximal body temperature elevations below 41.1 °C, 16 had temperatures between 41.1 and 42.1 °C, and 23 had temperatures above 42.1 °C. Mortality figures for these three groups—0 percent, 38 percent, and 61 percent, respectively—paralleled those of classic heatstroke, with higher temperatures associated with increasing degrees of multisystem damage and an unfavorable prognosis. This contrasted with findings in NMS as reviewed by Clark and Lipton (1984) in which body temperature exceeded 40 °C in only half of cases and 41 °C in less than 20 percent of cases. Furthermore, mortality rate across various temperature ranges in NMS were similar, suggesting that hyperthermia itself is seldom the major factor accounting for death in the NMS.

Both Bark (1982a) and Clark and Lipton (1984) noted that, in the absence of concurrent treatment with antiparkinsonian agents or heterocyclic antidepressants, neuroleptics involved in causing NRHS were more commonly those with greater degrees of peripheral anticholinergic activity, such as phenothiazines of the alkylamino group (chlorpromazine and promazine) and the piperidine group (thioridazine and mepazine). Cases of NRHS attributed to high-potency agents, such as the piperazine phenothiazines (perphenazine, trifluoperazine, and fluphenazine), as well as the butyrophenones (haloperidol)—all low in anticholinergic activity—involved concomitant treatment with anticholinergic agents in all but three reported cases: single cases associated with trifluoperazine, fluphenazine, and haloperidol. These findings suggest that anticholinergic-induced inhibition of sweating contributed to the development of NRHS in most instances. Still, those few reports of NRHS in patients treated solely with high-potency neuroleptics suggest that neuroleptics must be regarded as capable of causing NRHS independent of adjunctive therapy with anticholinergic agents or intrinsic anticholinergic effects of neuroleptics themselves.

Treatment and Prevention

Heatstroke is a preventable condition (Bark 1982b). All persons involved in the treatment, care, and supervision of psychiatric patients should be aware of the signs and symptoms of heatstroke and the need for immediate action. A complete discussion of the treatment of heatstroke is beyond the scope of this chapter; the interested reader is referred to reviews elsewhere (Anderson et al. 1983; Gross et al. 1983; Knochel 1980).

All forms of treatment aim at rapid cooling, fluid and electrolyte support, and management of seizures. In some cases, removing the patient from sunlight, removing the patient's clothing, wetting the body, and fanning to promote vaporization will be sufficient. However, most patients require intensive therapy, best rendered by a coordinated team in an emergency room setting (Anderson et al. 1983). Emergency departments in high-risk areas should have the potential to convert space into a "heatstroke room" with tubs, floor drains, and other special equipment necessary for the rapid management of heatstroke patients.

During summer heat waves, psychiatric patients must be protected from excessive heat and sunlight exposure, prevented from excessive exercise or physical labor, and encouraged to drink adequate amounts of fluid. Air conditioning probably represents the most effective means of preventing heatstroke. While neuroleptics are generally withheld following NRHS, in keeping with their role as a facilitator rather than a cause of heatstroke, they can generally be restarted with less concern about their danger in the absence of high environmental temperature or excessive endogenous heat production, unlike the situation that exists regarding restarting neuroleptics in recovered NMS patients.

A primary consideration in minimizing the risk of heatstroke should be the administration of neuroleptics in the lowest possible dosages. In the treatment of acute psychoses, rapid tranquilization and other "megadose" techniques now increasingly out of vogue should be employed with particular caution during hot summer days. The need for prophylactic or ongoing treatment with antiparkinsonian anticholinergic medication should be carefully evaluated. In addition, it is encumbent upon the treating physician to warn patients of the thermal risks of neuroleptics and to take particular note of patients at risk (e.g., agitated, poor judgement, indigent) in the heat.

Conclusion

Numerous clinical case reports involving neuroleptic-treated patients exposed to extremes of thermal challenge indicate that these agents can significantly impair thermoregulation. A consistent observation has been the tendency of neuroleptics to render patients thermally dependent on their environment, leading to hyperthermia in the heat. Similar findings have been reported in animal experiments across a wide variety of species. In the absence of human research data, animal studies form the basis for understanding the effects of neuroleptics on thermoregulation. The literature indicates that neuroleptics impair central thermoregulation in the AH/POA and other areas, and that this impairment appears to be mediated primarily through effects on CNS monoamine systems, particularly dopamine.

Suppression of central heat loss mechanisms by neuroleptics appears to be involved in the pathogenesis of both NRHS and NMS. However, in NMS, excess heat appears to be derived primarily from neuroleptic-induced extrapyramidal rigidity and possibly from direct effects of neuroleptics on skeletal muscle. In NRHS, excess heat is derived from a hot environment. Thus NMS appears to represent a genuine form of drug-induced heatstroke. In contrast, NRHS is best viewed as a drug-facilitated heatstroke in which neuroleptics increase vulnerability to a well-known form of environmental heat illness by interfering with heat dissipation. Among drug-related hyperthermias, NRHS most closely resembles classic heatstroke rather than exertional heatstroke. It appears likely that the anticholinergic effects of neuroleptics themselves, or anticholingergic agents often administered concurrently with neuroleptics, can facilitate NRHS. However, high-potency neuroleptics possessing little anticholingeric activity may be capable of causing NRHS when they are administered alone.

Chapter 3

Hyperthermia Induced by Other Psychoactive Drugs

Chapter 3

Hyperthermia Induced by Other Psychoactive Drugs

As discussed in the preceding chapters, data obtained from clinical and animal studies convincingly implicate neuroleptic drugs in disorders of thermoregulation, including neuroleptic malignant syndrome (NMS) and heatstroke. In addition to neuroleptics, other psychoactive drugs—including lithium, tricyclic antidepressants (TCAs), monoamine oxidase inhibitors (MAOIs), and sympathomimetic, psychedelic, and anticholinergic drugs—have been implicated in the development of rare hyperthermic and hypermetabolic syndromes. An NMS-like syndrome has also been reported in association with pharmacologic reduction of dopaminergic activity in patients with basal ganglia disease.

In this chapter, an overview of the clinical aspects and theoretical mechanisms of these rare hyperthermic syndromes is presented. Clarification of the clinical manifestations of these drug-related conditions is essential in determining their resemblance to NMS. Recognition of similar features would have clinical significance in terms of differential diagnosis and, conceivably, may broaden investigations of common pathophysiologic mechanisms.

Hypodopaminergic Syndromes

In recent years, several intriguing reports have come to light in which NMS-like conditions were described in patients treated with agents other than neuroleptics, which could directly affect activity in dopaminergic systems in the brain. Since these cases are unrelated to neuroleptic use per se, they are not, by definition, examples of NMS. However, these cases provide compelling evidence supporting the hypothesis that an acute alteration in central dopamine activity may be a primary etiologic mechanism in the development of NMS.

Henderson and Wooten (1981) first reported this phenomenon in a 50-year-old patient with Parkinson's disease who developed hyperthermia (40.4 to 40.6 °C), tremors, rigidity, tachycardia, diaphoresis, and hypoxia 2 days after treatment with carbidopa/levodopa, amantadine, and diphenhydramine was discontinued. Although the patient was also receiving haloperidol (15 mg) and lithium carbonate (900 mg) daily for mania, these investigators concluded that the reaction was a result of the potentiation of haloperidol-induced dopamine receptor blockade by withdrawal of dopaminergic agonists.

Subsequent reports have confirmed the observations of Henderson and Wooten (1981), that a syndrome consisting of mental status changes, severe extrapyramidal symptoms, autonomic disturbances, and hyperthermia may occur following withdrawal of dopamine agonists in patients with Parkinson's disease (Figa-Talamanca et al.; 1985; Friedman et al. 1985; Gibb 1988; Gibb and Griffith 1986; Hirschorn and Greenberg 1988; Sechi et al. 1984; Toru et al. 1981). Rhabdomyolysis with serum levels of creatine phosphokinase (CPK) as high as 50,000 IU has also been reported as part of this syndrome (Friedman et al. 1985). Furthermore, like NMS, it may be life-threatening; three deaths have been reported (Gibb 1988; Gibb and Griffith 1986; Sechi et al. 1984).

Most often, this reaction has been observed when carbidopa/levodopa was withdrawn from patients with Parkinson's disease because of lack of response, severe dyskinesias, or psychosis. In these cases, the duration of antiparkinsonian treatment ranged from 6 months to 10 years. The onset of the syndrome followed termination of drug therapy in 1 to 7 days. In some cases, anticholinergic drugs were discontinued along with levodopa and this may have potentiated an imbalance of neurotransmitters in the extrapyramidal system. However, in other cases, continuation of anticholinergics had little discernible effect on the evolution of the reaction (Burke et al. 1981; Gibb and Griffith 1986).

In addition to intensive, supportive care, treatment to date has usually consisted of reintroduction of dopamine agonists and anticholinergic drugs, although this pharmacologic strategy did not prevent a fatal outcome in three cases (Gibb 1988; Gibb and Griffith 1986; Sechi et al. 1984). In one case, dantrolene was used successfully in combination with levodopa and bromocriptine in the management of NMS-like symptoms (Figa-Talamanca et al. 1985).

In cases reported by Friedman et al. (1985) and Pfeiffer and Sucha (1985), a fatal NMS-like condition developed during "off" episodes in patients with Parkinson's disease while treatment with carbidopa/levodopa was maintained. While the exact mechanism underlying the on-off phenomenon is unknown, available evidence suggests that off periods correlate with troughs of plasma concentrations and striatal activity of levodopa (Quinn 1987). In the case reported by Pfeiffer and Sucha (1985), the reaction occurred in a patient who was also taking lithium (900 mg) daily, which had been prescribed in an attempt to ameliorate episodes of "freezing" associated with maintenance levodopa therapy (Reches and Fahn 1983). Noting the resemblance of the reactions in this patient to reports of hyperthermia related to lithium-neuroleptic combinations, Pfeiffer and Sucha (1985) suggested that lithium should be used cautiously in Parkinson's disease patients experiencing on-off fluctuations.

Similar reactions have been reported in patients with other pharmacologically induced reductions in dopamine activity. For example, Burke et al. (1981) reported a patient with Huntington's disease who developed confusion, hyperthermia, and severe dystonia after treatment over 7 months with tetrabenazine and alpha-methyl-tyrosine. Alpha-methyl-tyrosine specifically inhibits central and peripheral catecholamine synthesis by blocking tyrosine hydroxylase. Similar to reserpine, tetrabenazine depletes central stores of catecholamines, although a role for tetrabenazine in blocking dopamine receptors has also been proposed (Login et al. 1982). Haggerty et al. (1987) reported the development of "premonitory signs of NMS" in a patient treated with reserpine, who later developed the full NMS syndrome following treatment with neuroleptics. The chlorbenzamide derivative metoclopramide, which acts as a dopamine antagonist and is prescribed as an antiemetic, has induced an NMS-like reaction in several patients resulting in two deaths (Cassidy and Bansal 1988; Friedman et al. 1987; Patterson 1988; Robinson et al. 1985; Samie 1987; Wandless et al. 1980).

Pathogenesis

These cases demonstrate that, in addition to NMS, which is associated with neuroleptic-induced dopamine-receptor blockade, potentially life-threatening hyperthermic reactions may occur following administration of dopamine-depleting drugs, following withdrawal of dopamine agonists, or as a result of functional changes in dopamine activity during off episodes in Parkinson's disease. Thus inhibition of dopamine transmission, regardless of etiology, appears to be the common mechanism underlying these reactions.

Furthermore, since the neurodegenerative process in Parkinson's disease and systemically administered dopamine agonists and antagonists presumably affect the cortex, limbic system, and hypothalamus in addition to the basal ganglia (Alvord and Forno 1987; Langston and Forno 1978; Scatton et al. 1982), concurrent dysfunction in a number of dopamine pathways may be necessary for the development of NMS-like symptoms. In fact, inhibition of dopamine activity in mesocortical and mesolimbic tracts has been invoked to explain cognitive decline, autonomic dysfunction, and impairment of thermoregulation in Parkinson's disease (Appenzeller and Goss 1971; Elliot et al. 1974; Goetz et al. 1986; Gubbay and Barwick 1966; Tanner et al. 1987). While changes in other neurotransmitter systems—including norepinephrine, serotonin, acetylcholine, gamma-aminbutyric acid (GABA), and neuropeptides—have been reported in Parkinson's disease (Voigt and Uhl 1987; Wooten 1987), their clinical significance in relation to motor symptoms and hyperthermia remains unclear.

The development of animal models, which could be used to investigate dopamine-mediated hyperthermic syndromes, may be facilitated by recent reports of a parkinsonian state in substance abusers inadvertently exposed to 1-methyl-4-phenyl-1,2,3,6-tetrahydropyridine (MPTP) (Ballard et al. 1985; Burns et al. 1985; Kopin 1987). While attempts to induce parkinsonism using MPTP in rodents have not been entirely successful, administration of MPTP in primates has resulted in a profound parkinsonian state (Burns et al. 1983; Heikkila et al. 1987; Jenner and Marsden 1986; Langston et al. 1984). Although elevated serum CPK and diaphoresis have been occasionally reported (Ballard et al. 1985), hyperthermia and hypermetabolic symptoms have not yet been observed in humans or animals exposed to this neurotoxin. This is puzzling because the rapid onset of parkinsonism associated with destruction of dopamine-containing neurons by MPTP would seem to parallel the acute development of hyperthermia in susceptible patients treated with neuroleptics or withdrawn from dopamine agonists. However, MPTP-induced parkinsonism is unique; MPTP selectively damages dopamine neurons in the zona compacta of the substantia nigra whereas the neuropathology of idiopathic Parkinson's disease is multifocal and the effects of dopamine agonists and antagonists are similarly not limited to the nigrostriatal tract (Heikkila et al. 1987; Jenner and Marsden 1986). In addition, degenerative changes in other neurotransmitter systems reported in the idiopathic disease may not occur in MPTP-induced parkinsonism (Ballard et al. 1985; Burns et al. 1985; Heikkila et al. 1987; Jenner and Marsden 1986). However, transient functional changes in extrastriatal dopamine, and norepinephrine and serotonin, associated with acute behavioral effects reminiscent of the "serotonin syndrome" (Jacobs 1976; Jacobs and Kleinfuss 1975), have been reported after MPTP administration (Burns et al. 1983; Chiueh et al. 1984a, 1984b; Hara et al. 1987; Kopin 1987).

Thus further study of MPTP-induced parkinsonism may clarify the role of extrastriatal dopamine and other neurotransmitters, as well as systemic factors, in the development of acute hyperthermic syndromes. In general, investigations of animal models of hypodopaminergic states, induced by MPTP and other neurotoxins (Kopin 1987), afford the opportunity to examine, on an experimental basis, the conditions necessary for the development of NMS-like reactions.

Lithium

Neurotoxicity related to treatment with lithium has been recognized for many years. A broad range of effects on both central and peripheral components of the nervous system has been described (Jefferson et al. 1987; Sansone and Ziegler 1985).

In states of mild intoxication, vomiting and diarrhea may be accompanied by apathy, lethargy, weakness, and a worsening tremor. With more severe intoxication, an acute encephalopathy may develop, characterized by mental confusion, ataxia, dysarthria, gross tremor, choreoathetoid movements, myoclonus, parkinsonism, hyperreflexia, cranial nerve and other focal signs, seizures, coma, and death. Encephalopathy due to lithium toxicity is often accompanied by slowing of the dominant rhythm on electroencephalogram (EEG) (Sansone and Ziegler 1985).

A number of investigators have found that neurotoxicity may occur at serum levels of lithium in the therapeutic range, perhaps due to variation in sensitivity or relatively greater concentrations of lithium in brain tissue in some patients (Evans and Garner 1979; Jefferson et al. 1987; Lewis 1983; Sansone and Ziegler 1985; West and Meltzer 1979). In addition, it has been suggested that elderly patients, patients with underlying brain disease, and patients treated with other psychotropic drugs may be at risk for developing lithium neurotoxicity (Baldessarini et al. 1970; Johnels et al. 1976; Shopsin et al. 1970; Smith and Helms 1982).

While the mortality rate following serious lithium overdose approaches 15 percent (Hansen and Amdisen 1978; Schou 1984; Tesio et al. 1987), an additional 10 percent of patients appear to be at risk for irreversible neurologic damage (Prakesh et al. 1982b; Sansone and Ziegler 1985; Tesio et al. 1987). Most often, patients are left with cerebellar abnormalities and movement disorders, although changes in cortical functions, for example, diminished short-term memory (Apte and Langston 1983; Schou 1984), as well as evidence of peripheral neuropathy (Schou 1984) have been described. In a review of cases with neurologic sequelae, Schou (1984) found that some improvement could be expected 6 to 12 months after intoxication, whereas change was unlikely to occur after 1 year.

Hyperthermia, as reported in NMS, is not typical of lithium neurotoxicity, although lithium was associated with heatstroke in one case (Lowance 1980), and fever has been reported in comatose patients usually in association with intercurrent infection (Schou et al. 1968; Tesio et al. 1987). However, in four cases, fever was associated with lithium treatment in the absence of signs of infection or intoxication. Ananth and Ruskin (1974) reported the development of hyperthermia (39 °C), hypertension, transient extrapyramidal signs, urinary retention, and leucocytosis in a patient with a therapeutic lithium level. A patient reported by Gabuzda and Frankenburg (1987) developed a temperature of 39.8 °C on lithium 3 years after a similar episode of lithium-related fever occurred following recovery from NMS (Downey et al. 1984). Susman and Addonizio (1987) reported recurrence of NMS symptomatology in two patients treated with therapeutic doses of lithium just after recovery from NMS; the investigators noted that the proximity of neuroleptic exposure in these cases suggests that toxicity may have resulted from the lithium-neuroleptic combination rather than effects of lithium alone.

In addition to reports of encephalopathy, and rare instances of hyperthermia, a number of investigators have focused specifically on extrapyramidal effects of lithium. Shopsin and Gershon (1975) reported that 16 of 21 patients receiving lithium beyond 1 year showed evidence of mild cogwheel rigidity. They reported that this symptom was not responsive to antiparkinsonian drugs and suggested that the development and severity of rigidity correlated primarily with duration of treatment. Similarly, Branchey et al. (1976) and Kane et al. (1978) found evidence of extrapyramidal dysfunction in patients treated with lithium, although at a significantly lower incidence compared to the report of Shopsin and Gershon (1975). Branchey et al. (1976) found cogwheel rigidity in three of 36 patients and Kane et al. (1978) in two of 38 patients, and neither group of investigators found anticholinergic drugs to be particularly effective. Extrapyramidal symptoms in association with lithium therapy have been reported by other investigators as well (Asnis et al. 1979; Johnels et al. 1976; Sansone and Ziegler 1985; Tyrer et al. 1980). In all of these reports the extrapyramidal changes were mild, and the causal relationship with lithium may be complicated by prior exposure to neuroleptics (Jefferson et al. 1987). Nevertheless, these cases suggest that lithium may have clinically significant effects on the extrapyramidal system.

Conflicting data concerning extrapyramidal effects of lithium have emerged from clinical reports describing the use of lithium in the treatment of tardive dyskinesia. Although lithium has been reported to delay the development and reduce the severity of tardive dyskinesia (Gerlach et al. 1975; Reda et al. 1975), others have found that lithium exerts no significant effect on tardive dyskinesia (Foti and Pies 1986; Jus et al. 1978; Simpson et al. 1976; Yassa et al. 1984), or may even exacerbate the movement disorder (Beitman 1978; Crews and Carpenter 1977; Himmelhoch et al. 1980; Jefferson et al. 1987).

Similarly, there have been conflicting reports on the efficacy of lithium in the prophylactic management of "freezing" episodes in patients with Parkinson's disease maintained on levodopa (Coffey et al. 1982; Jefferson et al. 1987; Lieberman and Gopinathan 1982; Pfeiffer and Sucha 1985; Reches and Fahn 1983).

Finally, lithium affects the peripheral nervous system at therapeutic and toxic doses. As with central effects, peripheral toxicity may be enhanced in patients with preexisting neuromuscular disorders (Sansone and Ziegler 1985). Flaccid paralysis, proximal muscle weakness, fasciculations, and areflexia usually accompany lithium-induced encephalopathy. There have been isolated reports of myopathy (Julien et al. 1979) and myasthenia gravis-like illnesses (Dilsaver 1987; Neil et al. 1976) in lithium-treated patients. Rhabdomyolysis is unusual but was reported in a single case with many of the features of NMS (Unger et al. 1982). However, the role of concurrently administered drugs in this case was not entirely clear. Lithium appears to potentiate neuromuscular blockade by pancuronium and succinylcholine during anesthesia (Jefferson et al. 1987), perhaps by reducing acetylcholine synthesis at the nerve terminal (Vizi et al. 1972) or by down-regulation of acetylcholine receptors at the neuromuscular junction (Dilsaver 1987; Pestronk and Drachman 1980). Lithium has also been associated with the development of a reversible neuropathy (Brust et al. 1979; Newman and Saunders 1979) and the reduction of motor nerve conduction velocity (Girke et al. 1975).

In summary, lithium has diverse toxic effects on the nervous system at several levels. Following acute intoxication, a progressive encephalopathy may ensue with pronounced changes in mentation as well as cerebellar and motor functioning. Patients with prior evidence of neurologic dysfunction may be at increased risk for adverse reactions, even at therapeutic serum levels. In some patients, irreversible neurologic syndromes may persist beyond the phase of acute intoxication. Apart from secondary complications of acute toxicity, hyperthermia due to lithium is unusual, although it has been reported in a few patients, some of whom previously developed NMS after neuroleptic administration. Finally, changes in the extrapyramidal system resulting from therapeutic doses of lithium appear to be clinically infrequent and controversial.

Lithium-Neuroleptic Combinations

Lithium is often used in combination with neuroleptics in the treatment of mania. Although this combination has proven valuable and well tolerated by the majority of patients, there has been continuing controversy over the potential for synergistic neurotoxicity. Some investigators have reported that lithium potentiates extrapyramidal symptoms in patients concurrently receiving neuroleptics. For example, Sachdev (1986) reported the development of rigidity, tremor, and akinesia in a patient treated with fluphenazine decanoate after lithium was added. Addonizio (1985) reported two patients who tolerated treatment with neuroleptics but developed parkinsonian symptoms after lithium therapy was initiated.

A more severe form of neurotoxicity in patients treated with lithium and neuroleptics has also been described. Cohen and Cohen (1974) reported a severe encephalopathic syndrome arising in four patients during the course of treatment with haloperidol and lithium. As described by these investigators, this syndrome, which resulted in irreversible brain damage, consisted of lethargy, fever, tremors, confusion, and extrapyramidal and cerebellar dysfunction accompanied by leukocytosis and elevated serum enzymes, blood urea nitrogen, and glucose. They suggested that these reactions were unlikely to result from either drug alone and proposed that lithium and haloperidol acted synergistically on neuronal metabolic or membrane functions.

In response to this alarming report, a number of investigators suggested that these cases were artifactual, were due to factors other than drugs, represented inappropriate use of the drugs, or were explainable on the basis of toxicity of either drug alone (Jefferson and Greist 1980; Shopsin et al. 1976; Tupin and Schuller 1978). In addition, several investigators reviewed series of patients treated with combined medications and were unable to find examples of severe neurotoxicity. Small et al. (1975) evaluated the use of lithium combined with neuroleptics in 22 schizophrenic patients and reported that only one patient developed confusion and memory loss, although earlier studies suggested that schizophrenics were prone to develop signs of lithium neurotoxicity (Shopsin et al. 1970). Additional studies of combined therapy in schizophrenics or schizoaffective patients also failed to reveal unexpected toxicity (Biederman et al. 1979; Growe et al. 1979). Baastrup et al. (1976) reviewed records of 425 schizoaffective or bipolar manic patients treated with haloperidol and lithium and found that the combination did not seem to increase the frequency or intensity of side effects. Juhl et al. (1977) found no evidence of enhanced neurotoxicity in 55 manic patients treated with this combination. Abrams and Taylor (1979) and Krishna et al. (1978) reviewed clinical aspects and EEGs of patients treated with combined therapy and did not find evidence of enhanced neurotoxicity. Recently, Goldney and Spence (1986) conducted a retrospective study comparing 60 manic patients treated only with neuroleptics to 69 manic patients treated with neuroleptics and lithium. They found no differences between these groups in side effects and complications.

In contrast, Miller and Menninger (1987b) found evidence of neurotoxicity consisting of delirium, extrapyramidal symptoms, and ataxia in six (27 percent) of 22 bipolar patients treated with lithium and neuroleptics. In an expanded retrospective study, these same investigators reported the development of similar neurotoxic changes in eight (20 percent) of 41 patients receiving concurrent treatment (Miller and Menninger 1987a). Furthermore, unexpected and severe toxicity, sometimes resulting in persistent neurologic damage, has continued to be described in sporadic case reports of patients treated with lithium and neuroleptics (Addy et al. 1986; Alevizos 1979; Boudduresques et al. 1986; Coffey and Ross 1980; Destée et al. 1978; Donaldson and Cunningham 1983; Fetzer et al. 1981; Izzo and Brody 1985; Jeffries et al. 1984; Keitner and Rahman 1984; Loudon and Waring 1976; Mann et al. 1983; Menes et al. 1980; Miller et al. 1986; Prakash et al. 1982a; Sandyk and Hurwitz 1983; Sellers et al. 1982; Singh 1982; Spring 1979b; Standish-Barry and Shell 1983; Thomas 1979; Thomas et al. 1982; Thornton and Pray 1975; Yassa 1986). In a review of 39 case reports, Prakash et al. (1982b) found that 76.3 percent of such cases occurred in patients treated with neuroleptics and lithium for mood disorders, although in some cases schizophrenia and mental retardation were the principal diagnoses. In cases of toxicity attributed to the lithium-neuroleptic combination, women outnumbered men by a factor of 2 or 3 to 1. The ages ranged from 16 to 64 years, with a mean ($\pm$ SD) of 46 $\pm$ 12 years (Prakash et al. 1982b).

Haloperidol was involved in 67 percent of cases of combined neurotoxicity, but other neuroleptics that were implicated include fluphenazine, perphenazine, flupenthixol, thiothixene, chlorpromazine, and thioridazine (Prakash et al. 1982b). Prakash et al. (1982b) reported a wide range (63 to 32,500 mg) of neuroleptic dosages, expressed in chlorpromazine equivalents, with a median daily dose of 1,346 mg.

In reviewing 21 reported cases of combined neurotoxicity associated with haloperidol, we found that the mean ($\pm$ SD) daily dose of haloperidol (16.9 ± 12.8 mg) was well within the standard therapeutic range. Miller and Menninger (1987a, 1987b) demonstrated a correlation between neurotoxicity and the dosage of neuroleptic administered, although the dosages used were felt to be "suitable" therapeutic doses by these investigators. Similarly, in most cases, lithium dosing was within the standard range; in more than 90 percent of the cases the serum lithium level at the time of the reaction was below 1.5 mEq/l (Prakash et al. 1982b). Thus these reactions are not explained simply as a function of excessive dosing of either drug.

The manifestations of neurotoxicity in these cases reflect a spectrum of neuropathic features, including stupor, delirium, catatonia, rigidity, ataxia, dysarthria, myoclonus, seizures, and fever. Although Cohen and Cohen (1974) suggested that this acute encephalopathic picture did not occur with lithium or neuroleptics alone, this is clearly inaccurate, as some of these cases are indistinguishable from NMS. In fact, separation of these cases from NMS is often arbitrary. Many reviewers have included them among series of NMS cases such that 10 to 20 percent of reported cases of NMS have been associated with the administration of lithium in addition to neuroleptics (Caroff and Mann 1988; Kurlan et al. 1984; Levenson 1985; Pearlman 1986). This suggests that some cases of neurotoxicity attributed to combined therapy may actually represent cases of NMS with lithium playing a secondary role. Among reported NMS cases, in which lithium was co-administered with neuroleptics, we found no difference in sex, age, symptoms, and outcome compared to NMS cases associated with the use of neuroleptics alone (Caroff and Mann 1988).

However, in their review of 39 patients treated with combined pharmacotherapy and not diagnosed as having NMS, Prakash et al. (1982b) found that, unlike NMS cases, there was a predominance of women affected. Furthermore, while there were no deaths reported by Prakash et al. (1982b), there was a significant risk (11 percent of cases) of irreversible neurologic deficits. Persistent evidence of dementia has been reported in follow-up from 3 to 10 months in at least four cases (Cohen and Cohen 1974; Sandyk and Hurwitz 1983; Thomas 1979) and persistent signs of cerebellar or extrapyramidal damage were observed in these four cases and in additional cases followed for 5 to 24 months (Donaldson and Cunningham 1983; Izzo and Brody 1985; Mann et al. 1983; Sellers et al. 1982; Spring 1979a). By comparison, persistent neurologic sequelae in NMS survivors are less commonly reported (Anderson and Weinschenk 1987; Eiser et al. 1982; Rothke and Bush 1986; Shalev and Munitz 1986; Tenenbein 1986).

Thus, while some cases of combined neurotoxicity resemble NMS, other cases are comprised of features characteristic of lithium neurotoxicity (Hansen and Amdisen 1978; Sansone and Ziegler 1985; Schou, 1984). In fact, several cases of toxicity associated with combined therapy have been attributed to lithium alone (Brust et al. 1979; Donaldson and Cunningham 1983; Izzo and Brody 1985; Rifkin et al. 1973; Sellers et al. 1982; Thornton and Pray 1975; Tung and Swainey 1978).

Spring and Frankel (1981) proposed that two types of lithium-neuroleptic toxicity may occur, an NMS-like reaction associated with haloperidol and other high-potency neuroleptics, and a primarily lithium-induced reaction associated with phenothiazines, especially thioridazine. While a number of cases fit these two categories, many have features of both, suggesting that adverse reactions to combination therapy may form a continuum of neurotoxicity ranging from predominantly neuroleptic-induced to largely lithium-induced.

The intriguing and persistent question as to whether this drug combination produces synergistic rather than purely additive effects is difficult to answer solely on clinical evidence. As reviewed above, many patients have variable degrees of both lithium and neuroleptic toxicity. In addition, controlled epidemiologic data on the incidence of rare but severe neurotoxicity resulting from lithium or neuroleptics alone are too limited to determine whether combined treatment augments the possibility of a severe reaction to either drug. Thus the question of synergistic mechanisms may be resolved only through experimental investigations of pharmacologic and biochemical interactions between lithium and neuroleptics.

Pathogenesis

Clinical reports of neurotoxicity have stimulated the development of a number of experimental strategies designed to investigate potential interactions between lithium and neuroleptics. To date, there is no evidence of an interaction between neuroleptics and lithium on thermoregulation in animals (Clark and Lipton 1984). However, Shimomura et al. (1979) reported that a fatal hyperthermic reaction occurring after tranylcypromine administration in rats pretreated with lithium was inhibited by neuroleptics and possibly mediated by dopamine and serotonin. Some studies have demonstrated direct pharmacokinetic interactions between these agents, resulting in altered plasma levels (Jefferson and Greist 1980; Nemes et al. 1987; Rivera-Calimlin et al. 1978). However, other investigators have found no pharmacokinetic interactions between lithium and neuroleptics (Demetriou et al. 1979; Forsman and Ohman 1977; Smith et al. 1977). Secondary metabolic changes resulting from toxicity due to one drug (e.g., dehydration in NMS) could alter the absorption and excretion of the other. For example, patients developing NMS while on lithium may be at risk for developing lithium toxicity. This may occur because dehydration resulting from decreased fluid intake, sweating, and hyperthermia, and renal failure resulting from volume depletion and rhabdomyolysis, may elevate serum concentrations of lithium. In addition, other manifestations of NMS, for example, hypoxia and hyperthermia, which may cause brain damage, could act synergistically with lithium in the destruction of neural tissue.

Data relevant to the problem of lithium-neuroleptic interactions have also been obtained from studies of the influence of neuroleptics on intracellular lithium levels. There is some evidence that red blood cell lithium levels correlate more closely with side effects than plasma levels (Elizur et al. 1972; Hewick and Murray 1976). Several investigators have reported that combined treatment results in increased red blood cell levels and tissue retention of lithium (Elizur et al. 1977; Strayhorn and Nash 1977). Pandey et al. (1979) and Ostrow et al. (1980) demonstrated in vitro that phenothiazines, but not antidepressants or haloperidol, resulted in increased intracellular concentrations of lithium. Their data further suggested that cellular accumulation of lithium appeared to be caused by enhanced transport of lithium through passive leak diffusion. These findings were supported in a clinical study by von Knorring et al. (1982) in which patients on a combination of neuroleptics and lithium had significantly higher red blood cell/plasma lithium ratios than patients on lithium alone. As in the study by Pandey et al. (1979), haloperidol did not have the same effect as phenothiazines or thioxanthenes. Thus data on cellular transport of lithium provide a mechanism whereby combined therapy would augment lithium neurotoxicity, assuming red blood cell transport processes resemble those in neural tissue. This would explain cases of combined neurotoxicity involving phenothiazines in which acute effects of lithium and their sequelae predominate, consistent with the proposal advanced by Spring and Frankel (1981) that some of the reported cases represent lithium neurotoxicity primarily.

These mechanisms (i.e., enhanced intracellular transport of lithium) seem less relevant in clarifying the pathophysiology underlying cases in which hyperthermia and extrapyramidal symptoms predominate, particularly when associated with haloperidol. However, analogous to experiments focusing on lithium transport, Nemes et al. (1987) reported that concurrent lithium administration resulted in higher concentrations of haloperidol in red blood cells, plasma, and brain compared to administration of haloperidol alone. It is less clear whether these higher neuroleptic concentrations correlate with toxicity.

While specific mechanisms have not been elucidated, it seems reasonable to propose that adverse effects of lithium-neuroleptic combinations on the extrapyramidal system reflect synergistic actions on dopamine neurotransmission (Bunney and Garland-Bunney 1987). Engel and Berggren (1980) reported that lithium has neuroleptic-like effects, possibly through inhibition of presynaptic catecholamine synthesis. Flemenbaum (1977) reported that lithium, acting on both pre- and postsynaptic neurons, could inhibit in rats behavior that developed following administration of dopamine agonists. Reports of increased levels of dopamine metabolites in striatal but not other brain regions of rats chronically treated with lithium suggest enhancement of dopamine turnover or release (Eroglu et al. 1981; Fadda et al. 1980; Hesketh et al. 1978; Maggi and Enna 1980).

Other investigators have shown that administration of lithium produces no changes in (Reches et al. 1984) or decreases (Friedman and Gershon 1973) dopamine metabolites in the striatum. In a retrospective clinical study of eight patients with mood disorders, Linnoila et al. (1983) found that lithium appeared to decrease dopamine and its metabolites in all patients.

In studies of chronic lithium administration in animals, no effect of lithium was found on haloperidol-induced increases in dopamine metabolism in the striatum, nucleus accumbens, or frontal cortex (Meller and Friedman 1981; Reches et al. 1984). However, there is substantial evidence suggesting that lithium prevents the development of behavioral manifestations of neuroleptic-induced supersensitivity of dopamine receptors (Bunney and Garland-Bunney 1987). Studies of dopamine-receptor binding in rat brain using [³H]-spiroperidol suggest that lithium may block the development of supersensitivity in some dopamine pathways by inhibiting the increase in number of dopamine receptors (Pert et al. 1978; Rosenblatt et al. 1980), although not all studies have successfully replicated this finding (Bloom et al. 1983; Lal et al. 1978; Pittman et al. 1984; Reches et al. 1982; Staunton et al. 1982a, 1982b). Conceivably, lithium-induced inhibition of compensatory changes in dopamine receptor function could augment neuroleptic dopamine receptor blockade and increase the likelihood of neurotoxicity, at least during chronic treatment. However, the acute effects of lithium on dopamine transmission and on neuroleptic-induced changes in dopamine activity appear to be variable, and therefore difficult to reconcile with a consistent mechanism for understanding combined neurotoxicity.

Since administration of lithium alters a number of other neurotransmitter systems, especially enhancing serotonergic activity (Blier et al. 1987), it may be worthwhile to consider the effects of these neurotransmitters in producing synergistic toxicity when lithium is combined with neuroleptics (Bunney and Garland-Bunney 1987; Shimomura et al. 1979).

While studies of neurotransmitter and receptor function have been inconclusive, potential synergistic interactions of lithium and neuroleptics on intracellular mechanisms involving secondary messengers also merit consideration. For example, lithium has been shown in some studies to inhibit dopamine-sensitive adenylate cyclase in the caudate nucleus of the rat (Bunney and Garland-Bunney 1987; Stefanini et al. 1978). Geisler and Klysner (1977) found that inhibition of dopamine-sensitive adenylate cyclase in rat striatum was significantly enhanced when flupenthixol and lithium were combined as compared to when either agent was used alone.

In addition, increased recognition of the role of phosphoinositide metabolism in receptor mechanisms and transmembrane signaling suggests that this system may be worth examining in relation to combined neurotoxicity (Rasmussen 1986a, 1986b; Snider et al. 1987). It has been firmly established that lithium, at concentrations comparable to therapeutic levels, inhibits myo-inositol-l-phosphatase, resulting in significantly lower myo-inositol and raised myo-inositol-l-phosphate levels in the brain (Allison et al. 1980; Sherman et al. 1985). Although it is unclear whether this effect persists with chronic lithium treatment (Renshaw et al. 1986a, 1986b; Sherman et al. 1985), a reduced ability to form myo-inositol could seriously compromise neurotransmitter systems that depend on phosphoinositide metabolism (Renshaw et al. 1986b; Snider et al 1987). For example, the decrease of myo-inositol found in diabetic animals is thought to initiate a series of changes in peripheral nerves leading to the later development of irreversible functional and structural alterations characteristic of diabetic neuropathy (Greene et al. 1987).

Furthermore, investigations of the phosphoinositide system may be relevant since phenothiazines have been reported to stimulate or partially inhibit phospholipase C, depending on dosage, albeit in the micromolar range compared to nanomolar clinical levels (Walenga et al. 1981). Phospholipase C mediates the hydrolysis of inositol phosphate to diacylglycerol and inositol-1,4,5-triphosphate in response to extracellular receptor agonists (Rasmussen 1986a, 1986b). Thus co-administration of lithium and neuroleptics could result in synergistic effects on this messenger system, thereby altering neurotransmitter-stimulated calcium-dependent metabolic processes, and augmenting toxic effects of either agent.

In summary, the question of synergy raised by Cohen and Cohen in 1974 remains enigmatic and unresolved. There clearly have been rare but definite cases of a severe encephalopathic syndrome, sometimes with persistent neurologic damage, which has developed in patients taking lithium in combination with neuroleptics. These cases appear to represent a continuum of neurotoxicity, ranging from cases resembling lithium neurotoxicity to cases indistinguishable from NMS. Most studies of sample populations of patients treated with this combination attest to the rarity of this reaction, and suggest that if synergy occurs between these drugs, it occurs only under unusual circumstances in certain predisposed individuals. Laboratory studies support a mechanism whereby phenothiazine neuroleptics may facilitate the influx of lithium intracellularly and enhance the neurotoxicity of lithium. In contrast, no consistent action of lithium on dopaminergic or other neurotransmitter or second messenger systems has emerged that correlates with enhanced extrapyramidal effects of neuroleptics in the presence of lithium, or with the possibility that combined therapy with lithium may enhance the risk or severity of NMS-like hyperthermic reactions.

Amphetamines and Sympathomimetic Drugs

Amphetamines

The clinical and pathologic features of toxicity with central nervous system stimulants have been described in detail (Clark and Lipton 1984; Fischman 1987; Seiden and Ricaurte 1987). Administration of toxic doses of amphetamines and related drugs leads to a characteristic syndrome consisting of sweating, mydriasis, tachycardia, hyperactivity, and confusion, which may progress to hyperthermia, delirium, seizures, arrhythmias, shock, renal failure, disseminated intravascular coagulation, and death. Because of the prevalence of abuse of these drugs, it is important to be aware of the clinical manifestations of toxicity, and to contrast this presentation with NMS and disorders associated with other psychotropic agents. In addition, investigation of amphetamine toxicity may provide a broader picture of pharmacologic mechanisms underlying hyperthermic syndromes in general.

Hyperthermia is often found in relation to severe amphetamine toxicity (Clark and Lipton 1984; Sellers et al. 1979; Zalis and Pauley 1963). As reviewed by Clark and Lipton (1984), amphetamine-induced hyperthermia appears to reflect enhanced heat production in skeletal muscle. In support of this, fatal amphetamine-induced hyperthermia in dogs can be blocked by curare (Zalis et al. 1965). Increased heat production in skeletal muscle usually results from hyperactivity, agitation, or seizures. Increases in serum CPK as well as elevations in body temperature have been reported in the aftermath of convulsive activity (Belton et al. 1967; Wachtel et al. 1987). While increased motor activity due to locomotor stimulation or convulsions is typical, and probably accounts for heat production in most cases, some patients develop NMS-like syndromes characterized by extreme muscle rigidity. The development of rigidity may be centrally mediated, or rigidity may develop secondary to the loss of control of calcium-dependent contractile mechanisms in skeletal muscle as a result of an excessive rise in muscle temperature (Fuchs 1975).

For example, Chavanet et al. (1984) described a fatal case of amphetamine poisoning in which hyperthermia reaching 42.5 °C was accompanied by the development of generalized rigidity and cardiorespiratory arrest, although earlier in the course of this case, a temperature of 40 °C developed in association with irritability and agitation alone. Simpson and Rumack (1981) reported a case of toxicity due to methylenedioxyamphetamine. The patient presented with generalized rigidity, opisthotonus, tachycardia, and a temperature of 41 °C. Laboratory studies showed a leukocytosis, elevated CPK, and myoglobinuria. Earlier, Krisko et al. (1969) reported a patient who developed hypertonicity and dystonia in association with hyperactivity, agitation, coma, and fever (43 °C) following the ingestion of amphetamine, amobarbital, and tranylcypromine. However, the role of tranylcypromine in the development of rigidity and hyperthermia in this case must be considered as discussed in the section on antidepressants.

An even more acute picture, with similar clinical features, was reported by Kendrick et al. (1977) in five patients after intravenous administration of phenmetrazine or methamphetamine. Within 15 to 60 minutes after drug administration, these patients developed a syndrome characterized by chills, fever (37.6 to 40.0 °C), diaphoresis, nausea, vomiting, diarrhea, and myalgias. This progressed to shock, disseminated intravascular coagulation, rhabdomyolysis, myoglobinuria, and azotemia. Kendrick et al. (1977) ascribed the muscle necrosis and fever to the combined effects of sustained hyperactivity and insomnia along with a "pyrogen reaction" occurring following the injection of possibly contaminated material. Muscle rigidity apparently was not observed in association with rhabdomyolysis in these patients.

Some investigators (Davis et al. 1974; Sellers et al. 1979) have recommended use of neuroleptics to treat severe hyperthermic reactions associated with amphetamine toxicity, reasoning that neuroleptics may reduce agitation and possibly reverse amphetamine-induced peripheral alpha-adrenergic activation and vasoconstriction. Although neuroleptics could prevent decompensation in an agitated patient, the tendency of neuroleptics to impair the thermoregulatory response to a heat load, to increase heat production through rigidity, and to reduce heat loss by peripheral inhibition of sweating could override potential beneficial effects once hyperthermia supervened (Kosten and Kleber 1987). Chlorpromazine was administered to two patients reviewed by Sellers et al. (1979); one died shortly after treatment began, and the other survived but became obtunded and hypotensive after administration of chlorpromazine (Ginsberg et al. 1970). In contrast, Gary and Saidi (1978) reported the effective use of intravenous droperidol in treating a patient who developed a temperature of 42 °C following methamphetamine intoxication.

Cocaine

Hyperthermia appears to play a major role in fatal cocaine intoxication (Catravas and Waters 1981; Olson and Benowitz 1987). Loghmanee and Tobak (1986) reported the development of a fatal hyperthermic reaction associated with cocaine and alcohol abuse in a 20-year-old man. The patient presented with stupor, tachypnea, tachycardia, rigidity in the jaw and lower extremities, and a temperature of 42.8 °C. He subsequently developed respiratory arrest, seizures, and ventricular arrhythmias prior to cardiac arrest. Interestingly, this patient was previously diagnosed as susceptible to malignant hyperthermia of anesthesia, based on muscle biopsy results, and a documented family history of episodes of malignant hyperthermia during anesthesia. This history prompted the authors to consider the effects of cocaine on sympathetic and muscular activity, vasoconstriction, and thermoregulation as possible precipitants of episodes of malignant hyperthermia in susceptible individuals. Wetli and Fishbain (1985) also reported elevated temperatures in association with fatal intoxication presenting as an excited delirium in seven cocaine users with relatively low blood concentrations of cocaine. Symptoms included psychosis, violence requiring restraints, and hyperthermia (38.8 to 41 °C), eventuating in respiratory arrest and death. Other cases have been reported in which the intravenous, intranasal, or oral administration of cocaine resulted in hyperthermia associated with seizures, agitation, mutism, rhabdomyolysis, and renal, respiratory, or cardiovascular failure (Bettinger 1980; Krohn et al. 1988; Merigian and Roberts 1987; Roberts et al. 1984).

The association between cocaine intoxication and acute rhabdomyolysis apart from hyperthermia has recently been emphasized (Herzlich et al. 1988; Roth et al. 1988; Schwartz and McAfee 1987; Zamora-Quezada et al. 1988). Roth et al. (1988) reviewed 39 patients who presented with rhabdomyolysis after cocaine intoxication. These patients typically presented with agitation and myalgias. Sixty-two percent of patients had temperatures above 38 °C, and 33 percent had temperatures above 40 °C. Death was most likely to occur in patients with rhabdomyolysis who developed acute renal failure, liver dysfunction, and disseminated intravascular coagulation. Myonecrosis in these patients may result from the vasoconstrictive and ischemic effect of cocaine or by a direct toxic effect on muscle metabolism (Herzlich et al. 1988; Roth et al. 1988; Venkatachari et al. 1988).

Hyperthermia probably results from increased heat production due to muscular activity and seizures compounded by reduced heat dissipation due to vasoconstriction (Olson and Benowitz 1987). Catravas and Waters (1981) demonstrated that neuromuscular blockade by pancuronium effectively antagonized hyperthermia associated with fatal cocaine intoxication in conscious dogs. These investigators also found that the lethal effects of cocaine poisoning could be antagonized by hypothermia and chlorpromazine. Although the use of neuroleptics has been suggested in the treatment of cocaine poisoning (Olson and Benowitz 1987), their efficacy may relate to nonspecific sedation since the potent dopamine receptor antagonist pimozide, unlike chlorpromazine, had no effect in preventing lethality from cocaine in dogs (Catravas and Waters 1981).

Considering the clinical resemblance between some cases of cocaine intoxication and NMS, Kosten and Kleber (1987, 1988) proposed that rapid death in cocaine abusers represents a variant of NMS. They speculated that hyperthermia in cocaine abusers results from a relative decline in postsynaptic dopamine availability in hypothalamic and mesolimbic systems following a period of sustained dopamine stimulation during active cocaine use. Based on this hypothesis, Kosten and Kleber (1988) suggest that dopamine antagonists may be contraindicated in cocaine overdose and conversely, dopamine agonists may reverse this potentially fatal syndrome.

Fenfluramine

Finally, von Muhlendahl and Krienke (1979) published a review of toxicity due to fenfluramine, an amphetamine derivative used as an anorexic agent and in the treatment of autistic children. They reviewed 53 case reports of fenfluramine intoxication and found that hypertonicity, rigor, trismus, or opisthotonus were reported in 34 percent of cases, tachycardia was seen in 81 percent, sweating was frequently observed, and hyperthermia (37.6 to 42.8 °C) was seen in 25 percent of cases. In addition to hyperthermia, coma, and convulsions, the signs of nystagmus, hypertonia, trismus, hyperreflexia, excitation, and sweating characterized the clinical syndrome of fenfluramine intoxication. Three patients with temperature above 40 °C died. In one case, high plasma levels of intracellular enzymes detected 2 hours after drug ingestion were suggestive of muscle necrosis. Signs of intoxication occurred 30 to 60 minutes after ingestion and lasted several days, although in 90 percent of lethal cases cardiac arrest and death occurred within 1 to 4 hours after ingestion.

Manifestations of fenfluramine toxicity may reflect abnormalities in serotonergic mechanisms. Fenfluramine produces rapid release and inhibition of uptake of serotonin, resulting in long-term depletion of serotonin stores (Schuster et al. 1986; Sulpizio et al. 1978). Sulpizio et al. (1978) tested a variety of pharmacologic agents on fenfluramine-induced hyperthermia produced in rats maintained in a warm environment (25 to 28 °C). They concluded that hyperthermia results from increased serotonin activity, probably through release of serotonin from presynaptic stores because the hyperthermic response to fenfluramine was abolished by pretreatment with parachlorophenylalanine, cyproheptadine, and methysergide. In addition, they found that neuroleptics varied in the ability to antagonize fenfluramine-induced hyperthermia. Potent dopamine receptor blockers, such as pimozide and haloperidol, were inactive or enhanced hyperthermia, whereas less potent neuroleptics had a variable effect or, in the case of clozapine, completely antagonized the hyperthermic response. This effect of clozapine suggested to these investigators that clozapine has significant anti-serotonin effects and may act to preserve a balance of dopamine and serotonin in the brain.

In contrast to the variable effects of neuroleptics on fenfluramine-induced hyperthermia reported by Sulpizio et al. (1978), von Muhlendahl and Krienke (1979) cited studies on experimental amphetamine intoxication in animals (Davis et al. 1974) as a basis for suggesting that neuroleptics and adrenergic antagonists may be useful in treating fenfluramine toxicity.

Pathogenesis

In animals, amphetamines generally elevate body temperature, although this effect is variable and depends on experimental factors (including the species chosen for study and ambient temperature). Although there is substantial evidence implicating central dopamine pathways in the hypothermic response to amphetamines administered in a cold environment (Lee et al. 1985), the mechanisms underlying the hyperthermic response remain uncertain. Amphetamines may produce a peripheral thermogenic effect due to release of systemic catecholamines (Weis 1973; Zalis et al. 1967), which may be compounded by adrenergic-mediated inhibition of heat loss due to vasoconstriction (Clark and Lipton 1984). As discussed above, clinical and animal data suggest that stimulant-induced hyperthermia is a result of increased heat production by skeletal muscle associated with agitation, seizures, or rigidity.

However, the primary site of amphetamine action in triggering a hyperthermic reaction may be central; hyperthermia can be induced by cerebral ventricular injection and blocked by intraventricular administration of 6-hydroxy-dopamine (Clark and Lipton 1984). Furthermore, since alpha- and beta-adrenergic antagonists inhibit and TCAs enhance amphetamine-induced hyperthermia, this response may be mediated by the action of amphetamines in releasing norepinephrine. As noted by Clark and Lipton (1984), central administration of norepinephrine generally lowers body temperature in primates and other species, which reinforces the notion that the hyperthermic response to amphetamines may be due primarily to norepinephrine stimulation of motor activity rather than direct norepinephrine effects on central thermoregulatory mechanisms. However, Wirtshafter et al. (1978) reported that in rats maintained at room temperature, electrolytic lesions of the nucleus accumbens and olfactory tubercle antagonized amphetamine-induced hyperthermia but did not block amphetamine-induced hyperactivity. Similarly, Norman et al. (1987) and other investigators (Danielson et al. 1985; Feigenbaum and Yanai 1985; Grahame-Smith 1971a, 1971b) have found a dose-related dissociation between behavioral stimulation and hyperthermia in rats following amphetamine administration. Thus, the hyperthermic response to amphetamines may reflect direct effects on central thermoregulatory processes in addition to nonspecific changes in motor activity.

Amphetamines and related sympathomimetic drugs affect monoamine neurotransmitters other than norepinephrine, which may be implicated in the production of hyperthermia. In particular, the reinforcing and stimulant properties of these drugs appear to be related to an increase in dopamine activity due to potentiation of release and inhibition of reuptake of this neurotransmitter (Fischman 1987; Lee et al. 1985). Implication of dopamine in amphetamine-induced hyperthermia is suggested by studies in which hyperthermia was blocked by electrolytic lesions of the mesolimbic dopamine system (Wirtshafter et al. 1978), or by administration of dopamine antagonists or dopamine-depleting drugs (Ulus et al. 1975). In addition, Norman et al. (1987) recently reported that short-term pretreatment with neuroleptics resulted in increased sensitivity to the hyperthermic effects of amphetamine in rats studied at room temperature, perhaps reflecting the development of supersensitivity of dopamine receptors.

However, data suggesting the involvement of dopamine in amphetamine-induced hyperthermia conflict with evidence supporting the role of dopamine in mediating pathways that subserve heat dissipation and the development of hypothermia (Lee et al. 1985) (see Chapter 2). Perhaps the hyperthermic response is mediated primarily by norepinephrine derived from excessive dopamine (Przewlocka and Kaluza 1973). Otherwise, differences between studies in the dopamine-mediated effects of amphetamines on temperature may be due to differences in experimental procedures, including species differences, duration, dose, route, and localization of drug administration and ambient temperature (Lee et al. 1985).

Alternatively, the development of hyperthermia, rather than hypothermia, due to dopamine-mediated amphetamine effects may depend on the state of or changes in dopamine receptor sensitivity, different classes of dopamine receptors, reciprocal or feedback interactions between dopamine pathways, or the influence of dopamine on other neurotransmitter systems. For example, based on studies in which apomorphine, amphetamine, and dopamine produced hyperthermic reactions in rodents pretreated with haloperidol, reserpine, and serotonin antagonists, Yamawaki et al. (1983) and others (Danielson et al. 1985; Feigenbaum and Yanai 1985; Fjalland 1979a, 1979b; Frey 1975) proposed that dopaminergic agonists may activate two separate dopamine-related thermoregulatory pathways in the brain, one resulting in hypothermia and the other in hyperthermia. Yamawaki et al. (1983) further proposed that the latter mechanism is mediated by secondary activation of serotonin and is haloperidol insensitive. Although this model is highly speculative, it implies that under certain circumstances amphetamines could preferentially activate a dopamine/serotonin-mediated hyperthermic pathway that could be blocked by serotonin antagonists and enhanced by neuroleptic blockade of the haloperidol-sensitive dopamine hypothermia mechanism (Sulpizio et al. 1978).

Although the mechanisms underlying amphetamine-induced hyperthermia remain speculative, it may be worthwhile to compare this condition with other hyperthermic disorders. In particular, it is tempting to consider hyperthermia due to amphetamines as a pharmacologic model for "functional" cases of lethal catatonia (see Chapter 5). As in amphetamine intoxication, lethal catatonia develops more frequently in an agitated or hyperactive patient, although stupor and rigidity may be the presenting signs or may occur secondarily in some cases. Moreover, the psychotogenic effects of amphetamines have been proposed as a model for functional psychotic disorders, which may be mediated by dopamine overactivity and which may progress to lethal catatonia (Bowers 1987). Finally, neuroleptics have been suggested as treatment for both lethal catatonia and amphetamine intoxication (see Chapter 5).

In contrast, any relationship between amphetamine-induced hyperthermia and NMS is unclear and problematic. Some investigators have suggested that the pathophysiologic response to the enhancement of dopamine activity by amphetamine-like drugs may be a useful model for investigating mechanisms underlying NMS (Kosten and Kleber 1987, 1988; Norman et al. 1987). Acute treatment with neuroleptics results in a short-term, compensatory increase in dopamine synthesis, release, and turnover (Bunney 1984; Rupniak et al. 1986). Prior to the development of depolarization inactivation with chronic neuroleptic treatment (Bunney 1984), this may correlate with the onset of NMS symptoms during the initial phases of neuroleptic treatment. Accordingly, NMS may resemble acute dystonic reactions. Excessive dopamine activity has been implicated in the etiology of neuroleptic-induced dystonic movements (Rupniak et al. 1986; Tarsy 1983). However, pharmacologic mechanisms underlying dystonia and NMS appear to be different because NMS responds to dopamine agonists and is relatively refractory to anticholinergic drugs. Furthermore, enhancement of dopamine activity cannot explain the development of NMS-like conditions in patients deprived of dopamine due to dopamine-depleting drugs, or withdrawal of dopamine agonists in Parkinson's disease.

While dopamine overactivity in NMS seems unlikely, amphetamine-like effects may relate to the proposal of Schibuk and Schachter (1986), that NMS may result from excessive norepinephrine relative to dopamine activity. Similarly, Ansseau et al. (1980, 1986) suggested that NMS may result from an interaction between norepinephrine and dopamine systems. Finally, peripheral catecholamines may be significantly elevated in NMS and may contribute to the generation of heat (Feibel and Schiffer 1981), as proposed for amphetamine intoxication by some investigators (Weis 1973; Zalis et al. 1967).

In summary, amphetamine intoxication may result in hyperthermia associated with increased sympathetic activity, rhabdomyolysis, renal failure, seizures, disseminated intravascular coagulation, coma, and death. Patients may appear hyperactive and agitated or, less commonly, may develop muscle rigidity. Amphetamine toxicity must be considered in the differential diagnosis of lethal catatonia and NMS. Furthermore, amphetamine-induced hyperthermia may serve as a useful model in the investigation of lethal catatonia, whereas its relationship to NMS is unclear. In fact, neuroleptics have been recommended to control agitation and thereby prevent the development of hyperthermia in patients on amphetamines. However, neuroleptics probably should not be used after hyperthermia develops, as they pose an additional hazard to effective thermoregulation.

The mechanisms underlying amphetamine-induced hyperthermia are uncertain. While effects on motor activity, peripheral vasomotor tone, and catecholamine-mediated thermogenesis appear to be important, direct actions of amphetamines on neurotransmitters involved in central thermoregulatory mechanisms require further study. In addition, investigation of the concept of a balance between neurotransmitters, and the possibility of conflicting effects of dopamine on thermoregulation, merit further critical consideration in relation to mechanisms underlying hyperthermic disorders.

Psychedelic Drugs

Phencyclidine

Phencyclidine (PCP) was initially introduced as an anesthetic, but following reports of postanesthetic psychotic states, pronounced muscle rigidity, and seizure activity, it ceased to be marketed in the United States. Nevertheless, since the 1960s PCP has continued to be used as a drug of abuse and appears to be a unique psychoactive drug with diverse neurobehavioral effects, including depressant, stimulant, hallucinogenic, and analgesic properties.

Signs of PCP intoxication are dose related. At low doses, patients may show ataxia, slurred speech, numbness of the extremities, sweating, muscle rigidity, and signs of catatonia. Catatonic features, including staring and mutism, are characteristic of PCP and may account for the "dissociative" state or "sensory blockade" that has been described, similar to neurolept-analgesia. At higher doses of PCP, anesthesia, stupor, and coma may appear, accompanied by elevated heart rate and blood pressure, hypersalivation, sweating, fever, and convulsions.

In a review of more than 250 cases of PCP overdose, Rappolt et al. (1979) divided intoxication into three stages. Patients in stage I (serum concentration, 25 to 90 ng/ml) showed nystagmus, hyperreflexia, generalized spasticity, salivation, ataxia, myoclonus, and behavioral toxicity ranging from catatonic stupor, hallucinations, and disorientation to combativeness and violence. They recommended diuresis, acidification of the urine, and treatment with diazepam and propranolol during this stage. In stage II (serum concentration, 100 to 300 ng/ml), patients became stuporous and verbally unresponsive and developed hypertensive and tachycardic episodes. In the final stage (serum concentration, >300 ng/ml), patients were generally comatose. In addition to tachycardia and hypertension, tachypnea developed with the potential for apnea. "Board-like" muscle rigidity, myoclonus, opisthotonus, and seizures occurred. In stages II and III a potentially life-threatening "adrenergic crisis" or "dopaminergic storm" sometimes appeared 72 to 96 hours after drug ingestion. This manifested as a hypertensive encephalopathy or "malignant-type" hyperthermia. The authors advocated use of propranolol to prevent this from occurring.

McCarron et al. (1981a, 1981b) reported the results of an extensive survey of 1,000 cases of PCP intoxication. In agreement with results of Barton et al. (1981), they found that behavioral abnormalities, nystagmus, and hypertension were the most common manifestations of acute PCP intoxication. Violent and agitated behavior was more commonly observed than lethargy and stupor. Generalized rigidity was seen in 5.2 percent of patients and localized dystonia in 2.4 percent of cases. Hypothermia (6.4 percent) was more than twice as common as hyperthermia (2.6 percent). Rhabdomyolysis, occasionally associated with renal failure, was the most common serious medical complication of acute PCP intoxication (Barton et al. 1981). Serum CPK was over 300 IU in 70 percent of patients in which it was tested. Patients with elevated CPK were equally likely to be violent, agitated, or calm. The highest CPK was over 400,000 IU. McCarron et al. (1981a) divided neuropsychiatric manifestations of PCP intoxication into four major (coma, catatonia, toxic psychosis, acute brain syndrome) and five minor (lethargy, bizarre behavior, violence, agitation, euphoria) patterns. Among patients with coma, 50 percent showed generalized rigidity, 25 percent had hypothermia, and 8 percent had hyperthermia above 38.9 °C.

The clinical picture of PCP toxicity emerging from smaller series of cases is somewhat variable. Tong et al. (1975) reported two cases of PCP poisoning. In one of these cases, the patient became agitated and psychotic and then developed diaphoresis, flushed appearance, salivation, and writhing. He was found to have a temperature of 38.3 °C; irregular respiration; dyskinetic, purposeless motor activity; nystagmus; rigidity; and hyperreflexia. He was treated with diazepam and chlorpromazine to control agitation and recovered in 4 days. Liden et al. (1975) reviewed findings of PCP toxicity in nine cases. They found that peak symptoms developed in 2 to 4 hours. Symptoms generally subsided within 24 hours. Common features included drowsiness, nystagmus, hypertension, ataxia, miosis, hyperreflexia, and agitation. More severe cases showed depressed respiration, opisthotonus, hyporeflexia, seizures, and progression to coma. Hyperthermia was not reported. Corales et al. (1980) reported the difficulty in distinguishing PCP intoxication from head injury in two patients involved in motor vehicle accidents. Both patients had staring and mutism ("state of sensory blockade"), temperatures between 37.4 and 37.5 °C, muscle rigidity, hyporeflexia, and agitation during recovery.

In their review of drug-induced heatstroke, Clark and Lipton (1984) found two cases of PCP intoxication with temperatures above 40 °C. Three other cases were described with only mild temperature elevations and were associated with rhabdomyolysis. Thompson (1979) reported the development of seizures, hyperthermia, rhabdomyolysis, and renal failure in a patient with PCP intoxication. Jan et al. (1978) reported coma and hyperthermia associated with PCP abuse. Armen et al. (1984) reported three cases, one fatal, in which PCP intoxication resulted in agitation and combative behavior, severe hyperthermia (41.7 to 42.2 °C), respiratory failure, and coma. All three patients had rhabdomyolysis and severe liver necrosis. The authors compared these reactions to malignant hyperthermia of anesthesia and speculated that the marked temperature elevations could be related to the anesthetic properties of PCP. Consistent with this notion, ketamine, a related arylcyclohexylamine anesthetic, has also been associated with hyperthermia and has triggered episodes of malignant hyperthermia intraoperatively in patients with known susceptibility to malignant hyperthermia (Page et al. 1972; Roervik and Stovner 1974). This suggests that hyperthermia associated with arylcyclohexylamines may share some features with mechanisms underlying malignant hyperthermia.

Cogen et al. (1978) described two patients who developed PCP-associated acute rhabdomyolysis. A 21-year-old patient developed stupor and agitation, abdominal cramps, vomiting, "writhing tonic movements," myotonic contractions, and opisthotonus within 2 hours of a PCP overdose. He was found to have a temperature of 38.3 °C, nystagmus, and muscle tenderness. Laboratory examination revealed a serum CPK of 210,000 IU and myoglobinuria. A muscle biopsy showed nonspecific changes consistent with muscle injury on electron microscopic examination. The patient recovered within 1 week. Similarly, the second patient initially had abdominal pain, stupor, and hyperactivity, and was found to be febrile (38.3 °C), with pronounced dystonic reactions, muscle contraction, and rhabdomyolysis (CPK of 9000 IU), which seemed to respond to treatment with pancuronium. The authors concluded that muscle necrosis was directly related to dystonic and excessive motor activity in these patients. They cited evidence from Kuncl and Meltzer (1974), which demonstrated that denervation of motor never input prevented muscle damage in PCP-treated restrained rats. However, more recent work by the same group has shown that the PCP-restrained experimental myopathy could also be inhibited by adrenalectomy, adrenal demedullation, treatment with beta-adrenergic antagonists, and pretreatment with dantrolene (Ross-Canada et al. 1983). Furthermore, dantrolene diminished muscle damage but did not reduce locomotor activity or stereotyped behavior observed in rats treated with PCP. Thus the rhabdomyolytic effect of PCP may be multidetermined and dependent on catecholamine stimulation as well as motor never activity, both of which may contribute to muscle damage through the release of calcium in the sarcoplasmic reticulum (Ross-Canada et al. 1983).

Pathogenesis

Similarly, hyperthermia or hypothermia in cases of PCP intoxication may be multifactorial in origin. Hyperthermia may be related to seizures (Wachtel et al. 1987) or to the frenetic overactivity and combativeness of patients subjected to the sympathomimetic or stimulant properties of PCP. PCP has a propensity to affect muscle, resulting in heat generation and necrosis, possibly mediated by motor nerve activity, peripheral catecholamines, or more direct myotoxic effects of the drug (Meltzer et al. 1972; Ross-Canada et al. 1983). PCP increases oxygen consumption in rats in vivo, increases mitochondrial oxygen consumption in rat liver homogenates (Domino 1964), and appears to uncouple oxidative phosphorylation (Lees 1961), all of which may contribute to the peripheral generation of heat.

The central neurochemical basis of behavioral and thermoregulatory changes associated with PCP intoxication are unknown. PCP affects several neurotransmitter systems; it antagonizes excitatory amino acids, enhances noradrenergic and possibly serotonergic activity, possesses anticholinergic properties, and binds to a specific PCP-receptor that is shared with psychotomimetic benzomorphan opioids (Balster 1987; Johnson 1987). While the anticholinergic properties of PCP may impair heat loss and contribute to hyperthermia, other pharmacologic properties of PCP may play a role in thermoregulatory disorders associated with PCP and related drugs.

PCP has amphetamine-like behavioral properties and has been characterized as an indirect dopamine agonist. PCP has been reported to inhibit dopamine reuptake, facilitate its release, and secondarily affect dopamine synthesis and metabolism (Balster 1987; Johnson 1987). However, as in the case of amphetamines, it is difficult to relate enhancement of dopamine activity with the clinical development of hyperthermia, rigidity, and rhabdomyolysis, apart from drug effects on locomotor activity. In contrast, the dopamine agonist properties of PCP could be invoked to explain the more common development of hypothermia in patients intoxicated with PCP (Lee et al. 1985).

While PCP toxicity may present as an NMS-like syndrome comprised of hyperthermia, sympathetic activation, and striking muscle rigidity, the unique behavioral and pharmacologic properties of the drug may represent an intriguing pharmacologic model for exploring potential mechanisms underlying lethal catatonia due to functional disorders. The psychotomimetic effects of PCP are well known and have been likened to schizophrenia (Bowers 1987; Rappolt et al. 1979). In addition, the search for an endogenous ligand for the PCP receptor may provide important insights into the function of this receptor system and its relation to functional psychotic disorders and hyperthermic conditions as well.

Lysergic Acid Diethylamide

Interestingly, lysergic acid diethylamide (LSD), a psychoto-mimetic drug with pharmacologic effects similar to serotonin, produces hyperthermia along with other sympathomimetic effects in humans and animal species (Clark and Lipton 1984; Domino 1964; Gorodetzky and Isbell 1964). For example, Klock et al. (1973) reported eight patients who developed hyperactivity, psychosis, and sympathetic activation leading to coagulopathy, respiratory arrest, and coma. One patient presented with dystonia and four patients developed elevated temperatures (38.2 to 41.7 °C). Friedman and Hirsch (1971) reported a patient with a temperature of 41.3 °C, associated with psychosis and hyperactivity. Although hyperthermia in these cases may reflect extreme exertion, it also underscores the potential significance of serotonergic mechanisms underlying hyperthermic reactions (Frey 1975; Jacobs 1976; Yamawaki et al. 1983).

120

Antidepressants

Heterocyclic Antidepressants

In contrast to neuroleptics, hyperthermia due to TCAs used at therapeutic doses is virtually unknown. In cases associated with overdose, the more common response is actually a decrease in body temperature (Clark and Lipton 1984, 1986). However, Clark and Lipton, in their 1984 review, found four cases in which hyperthermia occurred: three with imipramine and one with protriptyline. All four patients died. In a later review, Clark and Lipton (1986) identified one case due to amitriptyline and six cases due to imipramine. Among the six patients who developed hyperthermia related to toxic doses of imipramine, four were under 10 years of age and three of these children died.

Among newer antidepressants, amoxapine, an N-desmethyl analog of loxapine, a dibenzoxepine antipsychotic, has also been associated with hyperthermia, rigidity, and rhabdomyolysis during treatment with therapeutic doses (Burch and Downs 1987; Lesaca 1987; Steele 1982) as well as when taken in overdose (Litovitz and Troutman 1983; Taylor and Schwartz 1988). Some of these cases have been considered examples of NMS (Coccaro and Siever 1985). However, unlike NMS, prolonged seizures that have occurred following amoxapine overdose may have contributed to heat generation (Wachtel et al. 1987). Furthermore, the relationship between hyperthermia, rigidity, rhabdomyolysis, seizures, and acute renal failure in these cases is inconsistent so that common mechanisms underlying these manifestations are unclear (Abreo et al. 1982; Jennings et al. 1983; Pumariega et al. 1982). Yet the resemblance of cases of amoxapine toxicity to NMS is not surprising because amoxapine and its 7-hydroxy metabolite possess potent dopamine-receptor antagonist properties in addition to effects on noradrenergic, serotonergic, and cholinergic systems (Coccaro and Siever 1985; Steele 1982).

Nomifensine, which is chemically distinct from currently available antidepressants, has both noradrenergic and dopaminergic properties with little effect on cholinergic activity (Coccaro and Siever 1985). This drug, which has been withdrawn due to the occurrence of severe hypersensitivity reactions, has been associated with hyperthermia in 1 to 2 percent of exposed patients (Ames and Youl 1983; Clark and Lipton 1986; Judd et al. 1983). Associated symptoms included chills, malaise, and myalgias, suggesting that elevated temperature resulted from an immune reaction rather than effects on central structures.

Hyperthermia has also been reported when heterocyclic antidepressants were administered in combination with other agents. Hyperthermic reactions to tricyclics have been reported in connection with the use of sympathetic amines during anesthesia (Janowsky et al. 1981). Tricyclics used in combination with neuroleptics have been associated with the development of hyperthermia in several cases (Clark and Lipton 1984, 1986). About 4 to 5 percent of NMS cases reviewed by Kurlan et al. (1984) and Addonizio et al. (1987) involved concomitant treatment with tricyclics. Several investigators have speculated that concomitant use of tricyclics may enhance the likelihood of NMS in patients treated with neuroleptics. For example, Schibuk and Schachter (1986) proposed that TCAs may produce a hyperadrenergic state that is then compounded by neuroleptic-induced dopamine-receptor blockade. They suggested that NMS may be the result of an imbalance in the norepinephrine/dopamine ratio. A similar hypothesis was proposed initially by Ansseau et al. (1980), although in a subsequent neuroendocrine study of an NMS patient these investigators found evidence that NMS may be associated with both alpha-noradrenergic and dopamine-receptor blockade (Ansseau et al. 1986).

Pathogenesis

The mechanisms accounting for TCA-induced thermoregulatory dysfunction, and hyperthermic responses in particular, are unknown. Tricyclics, especially imipramine and amitriptyline, have potent anticholinergic activity that could impair heat loss via decreased sweating and could contribute to heatstroke in conditions of excessive environmental heat or endogenous heat production (Clark and Lipton 1984; see section on anticholinergic drugs). Restlessness, agitation, and seizures occurring in some cases could produce an internally derived heat load. As in NMS, some patients with tricyclic intoxication manifest rigidity and hypertonicity, which could produce excessive heat in these patients. This was apparently true in a case of imipramine poisoning (Lee 1961), although other agents may have played a role in this case. Dothiepin, a thio analog of amitriptyline, has been reported to cause a syndrome indistinguishable from NMS with hyperthermia, rigidity, rhabdomyolysis, catatonia, and tachycardia (Grant 1984).

Although studies of the mechanism of action of antidepressant drugs in the treatment of depression have focused on adaptational changes in neurotransmitters and receptor sensitivity associated with chronic administration, the mechanisms underlying hyperthermic reactions may relate more to acute neurotransmitter effects following high-dose drug administration. Acute administration of TCAs is thought to result in increased synaptic availability of norepinephrine and serotonin secondary to reuptake inhibition and decreased catabolism (Blier et al. 1987; Heninger and Charney 1987). Changes in serotonergic activity may be particularly important in the development of hyperthermia. Although data on the effects of increased central serotonergic activity on temperature in humans are limited, cases of hyperthermia involving the administration of m-chlorophenyl-piperazine, etryptamine, and zimelidine, relatively specific serotonergic drugs, suggest that enhanced serotonergic activity affects thermoregulation in humans (Clark and Lipton 1986; Mueller et al. 1986; Simpson and Davidson 1983; Yamawaki 1986). Yamawaki (1986) found a dramatic decline in abnormally elevated levels of 5-hydroxyindoleacetic acid following the successful use of dantrolene and bromocriptine in an NMS-like episode that developed in a patient treated with amitriptyline. It is conceivable that enhanced serotonergic activity could produce alterations in muscle tone and activity (Jacobs 1976) as well as hyperthermia (Yamawaki et al. 1983) in some cases of tricyclic poisoning. By comparison, there have been no reports of hyperthermia in patients treated with desipramine, a relatively specific inhibitor of norepinephrine uptake, despite the widespread clinical use of this drug.

Data from animal studies provide further support for serotonergic mechanisms underlying TCA-induced abnormalities in thermoregulation. There is overwhelming evidence that a serotonergic pathway in the hypothalamus subserves the central mechanism for heat production (Grahame-Smith 1971a, 1971b; Myers and Waller 1978; Sulpizio et al. 1978). Vetulani et al. (1981) reported that chronic electroconvulsive shocks augmented the hyperthermic response of rats to a serotonin agonist, and concomitantly produced an increase in the density of serotonin$_2$ binding sites. Goodwin and Green (1985) and Goodwin et al. (1985) reported that the hypothermic response in mice to a selective serotonin$_{1a}$ receptor agonist, which may act to decrease serotonin release via presynaptic receptors, was attenuated by chronic treatment with TCAs, MAOIs, and electroconvulsive shocks.

The evidence suggesting involvement of dopamine in TCA-induced hyperthermia is less clear. Although there are no data indicating consistent effects of TCAs on dopamine synthesis, turnover, or receptor binding, neurophysiologic and behavioral studies in animals have suggested that subsensitivity of presynaptic dopamine autoreceptors and augmentation of postsynaptic dopamine agonist effects develop following long-term TCA administration (Heninger and Charney 1987; Towell et al. 1986; Willner 1983). Overall, these delayed effects would enhance dopamine transmission, which could lead to hyperthermia by mechanisms analogous to those underlying amphetamine-induced hyperthermia.

Conversely, Towell et al. (1986) reported that brief treatment with desipramine appeared to enhance the effect of apomorphine on a behavioral measure of dopamine autoreceptor function, which would produce a diminution in dopamine activity.

Alternatively, TCAs may affect dopamine systems indirectly through changes in norepinephrine and serotonin systems, which may serve a neuromodulatory role in the release and activity of dopamine. For example, Russell et al. (1987) reported that chronic treatment with desipramine, but not mianserin or citalopram, attenuated alpha-2-adreno-receptor-mediated inhibition of dopamine release in the rat nucleus accumbens while not affecting beta-adrenoreceptor-mediated enhancement of dopamine release. In addition, serotonin-containing neurons, which originate in the brainstem raphe nuclei and project to the substantia nigra and basal ganglia, can alter the release of dopamine from terminals within the rat striatum (Chesselet 1984; Voigt and Uhl 1987). Potent serotonergic TCAs have been shown to inhibit the dopamine-mediated effects of apomorphine on contralateral turning in rats with unilateral lesions of the substantia nigra (Delini-Stula and Vassout 1979). Furthermore, hypothermia induced by high doses of apomorphine is antagonized by antidepressants, as well as adrenergic and serotonergic stimulants, and potentiated by the administration of serotonin antagonists (Menon and Vivonia 1981; Puech et al. 1981).

Monoamine Oxidase Inhibitors

MAOIs taken in overdose or in combination with other drugs have been associated with hyperthermia. In their review, Clark and Lipton (1984) identified one case associated with nialamide and two with tranylcypromine. Rigidity was described in one patient treated with tranylcypromine, and the other two patients were described as sweating profusely. All three died. In a later review (Clark and Lipton 1986), an additional two cases of hyperthermia were reported in patients who overdosed on phenelzine. Hyperthermia, also associated with rigidity and sweating following an overdose of tranylcypromine, was reported by Robertson (1972).

Recently, Kaplan et al. (1986) reported a case of phenelzine overdose in which signs of a hypermetabolic crisis indistinguishable from NMS or malignant hyperthermia were observed. In addition, their patient responded dramatically following administration of dantrolene. Similarly, Verilli et al. (1987) reported resolution of an NMS-like hypermetabolic state 1 day after administration of dantrolene in a patient treated with phenelzine. Cohen et al. (1987) reported a fatal case of "nonneuroleptic malignant syndrome" in a patient treated with phenelzine.

Toxic reactions to treatment with MAOIs in combination with other substances have been described. While ingestion of foods containing high concentrations of tyramine is known to cause dangerous hypertensive crises in patients on MAOIs, hyperthermic reactions have also been reported. Mirchandain and Reich (1985) reported the development of rigidity, mental status changes, and hyperthermia (42.1 to 44.4 °C) leading to death in a 26-year-old woman who ate cheese and drank wine while on therapeutic doses of tranylcypromine. Haloperidol and dantrolene were included as therapy but were not effective. Linden et al. (1984) reported the development of hyperthermia, tremors, rigidity, and rhabdomyolysis following a fatal overdose involving phenelzine and wine. Similarly, Brown (1970) reported hyperthermia, rigidity, coma, and hypertension in a patient who overdosed on phenelzine, aspirin, and wine. In this case, muscle relaxation following succinylcholine administration led to a rapid recovery. Zetin et al. (1987) reported similar findings in a patient on phenelzine who began a powdered protein diet. Brennan et al. (1988) reported a fatal NMS-like reaction in a patient treated with therapeutic doses of phenelzine, lithium, tryptophan, and benzodiazepines.

Toxicity involving hyperthermia has also been reported with MAOIs in combination with neuroleptic, amphetamine, and salicylate intoxication (Clark and Lipton 1986). The concurrent use of indirect acting sympathomimetic agents, for example, amphetamine (Lewis 1965), entails greater risks than direct acting agents, for example, norepinephrine, because the former rely on presynaptic neuronal stores that are excessive in MAOI-treated patients.

Narcotic-analgesics, especially meperidine, when administered to patients taking an MAOI, may result in severe hyperthermic reactions associated with agitation, hypertension, rigidity, and convulsions (Clark and Lipton 1984, 1986; Janowsky et al. 1981; Palmer 1960). The hyperthermic reaction to MAOI-meperidine combinations has been attributed to the release of serotonin because this reaction can be blocked in animals pretreated with inhibitors of serotonin synthesis (Janowsky et al. 1981; Rogers 1971; Rogers and Thornton 1969).

Pathogenesis

In all MAOI-related hyperthermic reactions, heat generation due to rigidity, restlessness, or seizures appears to be increased; heat loss mechanisms appear to remain intact. Presumably, as with tricyclics, an increase in monoamines may contribute to the development of rigidity and excessive heat production. MAOIs act initially to increase concentrations of several monoamines, including norepinephrine, serotonin, dopamine, and phenylethylamine. To date, hyperthermic reactions have been reported with MAOIs that nonselectively affect both major monoamine oxidase isoenzymes. With the development of highly selective MAOIs that inhibit only one form of the enzyme, it may become possible to distinguish the isoenzyme and neurotransmitter substrate associated with the development of hyperthermia. However, among the transmitters affected by nonspecific MAOIs, serotonin may be particularly important to consider in relation to mechanisms underlying these reactions (Blier et al. 1987; Myers and Waller 1978).

In fact, it may be productive to compare adverse reactions to MAOIs with the "serotonin syndrome" comprised of neuromuscular symptoms (myoclonus, tremor, rigidity, head shaking, and hyperactivity) and autonomic signs (salivation, skin flushing, diarrhea, and piloerection), which has been described in animals after administration of compounds that increase synaptic serotonin or directly stimulate postsynaptic serotonin receptors (Jacobs 1976; Jacobs and Kleinfuss 1975). Several cases of a condition, which has been compared to the serotonin syndrome described in animals, have been reported in patients treated with a combination of tryptophan and MAOIs (Lieberman et al. 1986; Pope et al. 1985). Interestingly, Price et al. (1986) recently reported the development of episodes of hyperventilation, diaphoresis, shivering, hyperthermia (38.5 °C), hypertonicity, and hyperreflexia in a patient following the addition of tryptophan to a therapeutic regimen of lithium carbonate and tranylcypromine and a similar case was reported by Brennan et al. (1988). As stated previously, administration of tranylcypromine has been associated with a fatal hyperthermic reaction in rats pretreated with lithium (Shimomura et al. 1979). This reaction was attributed to enhancement of dopamine and serotonin activity. Serotonin was also implicated in earlier studies in which tryptophan loading resulted in hyperactivity and hyperthermia in rats pretreated with tranylcypromine (Grahame-Smith 1971a, 1971b).

Moreover, the frequent occurrence of rigidity in MAOI-related hyperthermic episodes suggests that a hypothesis proposed by Lieberman et al. (1985) to explain neuromuscular effects of MAOIs is worth examining. This model is based on a hypothetical balance between serotonergic and dopaminergic systems affecting spinal cord mechanisms. Lieberman et al. (1986) suggested that an increase in serotonergic tone produced by MAOIs decreases central tonic inhibition by dopamine of spinal neurons, leading to alpha-motor neuron excitation and skeletal muscle activation. Serotonin excites motor neurons in the spinal cord whereas dopamine is inhibitory. Thus the increased serotonergic tone from MAOIs upsets the balance, resulting in motor neuron excitation. According to this model, neuroleptic antagonism of dopamine would also alter the serotonin/dopamine balance, resulting in motor neuron excitation, muscle activity, rigidity, and heat production.

MAOI-TCA Combinations

The clinical evidence concerning the efficacy and toxicity of MAOIs and TCAs used in combination has been examined in several comprehensive reviews (Lader 1983; Marley and Wozniak 1983; White and Simpson 1981, 1984). Uncontrolled clinical series involving at least 868 patients treated with a variety of MAOIs and TCAs have been reported (White and Simpson 1981). Severe and fatal reactions were not reported in these series. Generally, the authors considered side effects to be similar in nature, frequency, and severity to those observed with single-drug therapy. The most common problems were orthostatic hypotension and weight gain.

There have been a few controlled studies designed to test the relative advantages and risks of combined treatment. Davidson et al. (1978) randomly assigned 19 medication-resistant depressed inpatients to treatment with electroconvulsive therapy or a combination of amitriptyline and phenelzine. Although no serious reactions occurred among the drug-related patients, side effects led to dose reduction in four cases. Young et al. (1979) conducted a randomized, double-blind study in which 135 depressed outpatients who were not specifically drug resistant were assigned to treatment with phenelzine, isocarboxazid, trimipramine, phenelzine plus trimipramine, or isocarboxazid plus trimipramine. Combined drug treatment did not produce severe untoward effects. White et al. (1980) randomly assigned 30 depressed inpatients to open treatment with amitriptyline, tranylcypromine, or the combination of the two in reduced dosages. The three treatments resulted in equivalent therapeutic effects without any severe reactions. Finally, Razani et al. (1983) reported the results of a prospective, randomized, double-blind trial comparing the combination of tranylcypromine and amitriptyline to treatment with either agent alone in 60 patients who were divided among the three treatment groups and who met DSM-III (American Psychiatric Association 1980) criteria for major depression. All three groups improved equally and no instances of hypertensive or hyperthermic crises were noted.

In a recent retrospective study of 94 patients treated with tricyclics in combination with tranylcypromine and trifluoperazine, Schmauss et al. (1986) reported that side effects were similar to those resulting from the use of single drugs, although a hypertensive crisis developed in one patient. In another retrospective review of 207 patients treated with the fixed combination of tranylcypromine/trifluoperazine and either amitriptyline or clomipramine, Oefele et al. (1986) found significant toxicity in 12 (24.5 percent) cases when tranylcypromine/trifluoperazine was combined with clomipramine. Three patients developed hyperthermia up to 40 °C along with gross tremor; three developed a toxic delirium; four had unstable blood pressure, sweating, and tremor; one patient had hypertension and tachycardia; and one developed severe agitation. There was no relation between toxicity and drug plasma levels or doses, which were therapeutic in all cases.

Collectively, these uncontrolled and controlled studies support the impression of the relative safety of the MAOI-TCA combination when used strictly in accordance with recommended guidelines. Guidelines vary but most authors agree that adding a tricyclic to an established MAOI regimen may be especially hazardous. In addition, a 7- to 10-day washout period between switching drugs is recommended, although an even longer interval is desirable (White and Simpson 1984). Preferably, both drugs should be started at low doses with gradual increments. It has been suggested that potent serotonin reuptake inhibitors—and specifically imipramine, clomipramine, and tranylcypromine—may be particularly dangerous when used in combinations.

Examination of the reported cases of severe toxicity due to the MAOI-TCA combination reveals a range of clinical findings. The typical manifestations differ significantly from typical hypertensive crises and generally include an agitated delirium, which may progress to generalized hypertonicity, seizures, hyperthermia (to 43.2 °C), tachycardia, tachypnea, coma, and death (Lader 1983; White and Simpson 1981). This picture may be similar to NMS and lethal catatonia in some cases. It is also indistinguishable from the manifestations of overdose due to MAOIs or TCAs alone, which has prompted some authors to suggest that the combination is no more toxic than single drug therapy. However, in a few cases, a severe neurotoxic reaction developed in patients taking modest, therapeutic doses of both agents, leaving open the possibility that a synergistic effect may occur (Ayd 1961; Brachfeld et al. 1963; Davies 1960; Graham et al. 1982; McCurdy and Kane 1964; Oefele et al. 1986; Singh 1960).

Apart from attempted suicide by overdose, many of the reports of toxic reactions associated with the combination are complicated by concurrent use of other drugs, dietary indiscretion leading to tyramine reactions, coexistent medical conditions, and parenteral drug administration (White and Simpson 1981). Nevertheless, substantial clinical data from numerous case reports indicate that TCAs added to or substituted for treatment with MAOIs can provoke a severe and potentially fatal reaction.

Pathogenesis

The pathophysiology of these reactions is unclear. On a clinical level, agitation, restlessness, and seizures related to overdose may contribute to the development of hyperthermia. However, a number of cases were characterized by rigidity, diaphoresis, and autonomic signs reminiscent of NMS. Some of these cases actually involved concurrent treatment with neuroleptics and may represent true NMS (Babiak 1961; Bowen 1964; Hills 1965; Oefele et al. 1986; Peebles-Brown 1985), although other cases involving antidepressants alone also manifested rigidity and other features similar to NMS (Brachfeld et al. 1963; Ciocatto et al. 1972; Graham et al. 1982; Marra et al. 1965; Ritchie 1983; White and Simpson 1981). Richards et al. (1987) recently reported the development of a typical NMS-like hypermetabolic state in a depressed woman following an overdose with tranylcypromine, clomipramine, trazodone, cyclizine, and oxazepam. Temperature and rigidity decreased rapidly following treatment with the muscle relaxants pancuronium, diazepam, and dantrolene.

In a series of experiments with dogs, Himwich (1962) and Himwich and Peterson (1961a, 1961b) found that some animals developed hyperthermia after a single injection of tranylcypromine following a 5-day course of intramuscular imipramine. The mechanisms of hyperthermia appeared to be related to muscle activity and hypertonicity since it was completely blocked by curarization, although light barbiturate anesthesia also attenuated this response.

The pharmacologic effects of the MAOI-TCA combination have also been investigated in other animal species (Lader 1983; Marley and Wozniak 1983; White and Simpson 1981). Rabbits appear particularly sensitive, developing a hyperexcitable-hyperthermic syndrome leading to seizures and death following the administration of the MAOI-TCA combination (Loveless and Maxwell 1965). Elevated levels of serotonin were implicated in studies by Gong and Rogers

(1973), in which elevations of brain serotonin and the toxic reaction itself were prevented by premedication with parachlorophenylalanine. In rats and mice, the MAOI-TCA combination can provoke a syndrome of hyperactivity, tremors, and stereotyped behaviors. Similar to results with rabbits, studies using selective serotonin uptake inhibitors, parachlorophenylalanine, and tryptophan underscore the role of serotonin in these reactions (White and Simpson 1981).

Due to the diversity of animal studies, it is difficult to draw conclusions relevant to clinical toxicity. The nature of behavioral and physiological reactions in different species is variable. Most animal studies involved parenteral administration of relatively large doses of drugs. In addition, use of control groups exposed to equivalent doses of single drugs was limited. However, there are some parallels to the syndrome that occurs in humans (e.g., the relative potency and sequence of drugs producing toxic reactions). While clinical correlations must be considered cautiously in view of methodological limitations, the available evidence in some animal species implicates elevated activity of serotonin in the development of hyperthermic reactions to combined MAOI-TCA therapy (White and Simpson 1981).

In summary, there are rare cases in which antidepressants, used alone or in combinations, produced a syndrome similar to NMS. These are important to acknowledge from the standpoint of differential diagnosis. Furthermore, investigation of toxicity due to antidepressants may add to knowledge of mechanisms underlying hypermetabolic conditions. As in NMS, hyperthermia associated with antidepressants appears to result primarily from excessive heat production in muscle, although anticholinergic-mediated inhibition of peripheral heat loss mechanisms may contribute to hyperthermia in TCA-related cases. This implies that muscle relaxation, achieved by administration of dantrolene or other drugs, may be therapeutic regardless of the initial triggering agent (Kaplan et al. 1986; Ritchie 1983; Verilli et al. 1987; Yamawaki 1986).

In addition, hyperthermic syndromes due to antidepressants provide additional data supporting the role of serotonin in the development of clinical disorders of thermoregulation. Moreover, studies of antidepressant toxicity support the concept proposed by several investigators that NMS and related conditions may develop as a result of an interaction or imbalance in the activity of neurotransmitters involved in thermoregulation (Ansseau et al. 1980, 1986; Graham et al. 1982; Lieberman et al. 1985; Schibuk and Schachter 1986; Yamawaki et al. 1983). In particular, the hypothesis of a critical relationship between serotonin and dopamine, which affects thermoregulatory, autonomic, and neuromuscular function, may be worthwhile to consider as a basis for future investigations.

Anticholinergic Drugs

A number of drugs used in clinical psychopharmacology possess significant anticholinergic activity. Antiparkinsonian agents, TCAs, and low-potency phenothiazines act as muscarinic antagonists and may elevate body temperature either as a result of inhibition of cholinergic effects on central thermoregulatory mechanisms (Lin et al. 1980) or due to interference with peripheral heat loss by inhibiting sweating (Baldessarini 1985). In fact, use of atropine and related agents has been associated with compromise of thermoregulation in hot environments (Clark and Lipton 1984; Cullumbine and Miles 1956) and are considered as risk factors for heatstroke (see Chapter 2). However, in experimental studies of the effects of atropine in healthy subjects exercising or exposed to heat, body temperature did not rise to dangerous levels. Inhibition of sweating was no more than 50 percent, resulting in only partial impairment of heat loss mechanisms. This led Clark and Lipton (1984) to conclude that therapeutic doses of atropine are not likely to cause significant hyperthermia, at least in healthy subjects in thermally neutral environments, and that in order for hyperthermia to develop in patients, overdosage, an excessive heat load, or further inhibition of heat loss perhaps through central mechanisms would be necessary.

Intoxication with anticholinergics results in a well-described syndrome of atropinic poisoning that is characterized by central and peripheral signs (e.g., dry mouth, flushed dry skin, dilated pupils, blurred vision, tachycardia, urinary retention, and intestinal paralysis), which may progress to ataxia, hyperactivity, agitation, increased muscle tone, delirium, and coma. In a survey of cases of anticholinergic poisoning, Shader and Greenblatt (1971) found temperatures above 37.7 °C in 18 percent of adults and 25 percent of children. Temperatures above 40 °C are less common (Clark and Lipton 1984). In the absence of external heat stress in these cases, Clark and Lipton (1984) speculated that agitation and delirium resulting from toxic doses may have contributed to hyperthermia by the endogenous generation of heat.

Because of the pronounced signs of anticholinergic toxicity in the periphery, the inhibition of sweating, and the uncommon appearance of severe temperature elevations and rigidity, hyperthermia due to anticholinergic intoxication is unlikely to be mistaken for NMS. This is important because treatment may differ; physostigmine serves as a specific antidote in atropine poisoning but has no effect in NMS (Krull and Risse 1986; Patel and Bristow 1987).

Anticholinergics are often used in psychiatry in combination with other agents, including neuroleptics and antidepressants. As a result, their inhibitory effect on sweating may contribute to the emergence of hyperthermia due to thermoregulatory effects of other drugs used concurrently. For example, up to 23 percent of cases of NMS have developed when anticholinergic antiparkinsonian drugs were administered with neuroleptics (Kurlan et al. 1984), and nearly half of NMS cases involved treatment with either antiparkinsonian or TCA agents (Levenson 1985). Thus anticholinergics may contribute to heat stress when hyperthermia develops in association with neuroleptics or other drugs.

Conclusion

The clinical manifestations of NMS, including hyperthermia, rigidity, and autonomic and mental status changes, comprise a hypermetabolic syndrome that is not specific for this neuroleptic-induced disorder. These clinical features may be found in association with a broad range of systemic and local disorders affecting brain function. Diverse pharmacologic agents, including a number of psychoactive drugs, which may affect thermoregulation by a variety of proposed mechanisms, have been associated with NMS-like syndromes. Recognition of the nonspecificity of NMS symptoms and familiarity with the disease processes and drugs that have been associated with these symptoms are essential in the management of patients presenting with hyperthermic and hypermetabolic syndromes. In addition, examination of the spectrum of drugs associated with NMS-like conditions provides a rationale to expand investigations of the theoretical mechanisms underlying these disorders.

Several cases have now been reported in which abrupt withdrawal of dopamine agonists from patients treated for Parkinson's disease resulted in hyperthermic reactions indistinguishable from NMS. In addition to data on NMS-like reactions in patients treated with dopamine-depleting drugs or experiencing "freezing" episodes during levodopa administration, these reactions add clinical support to the hypothesis implicating hypodopaminergic activity as a primary mechanism underlying the development of NMS. The clinical evidence also suggests that a pharmacologic model of NMS involving selective destruction or inhibition of dopamine pathways by neurotoxins could be developed. Such a model, based on the hypodopaminergic hypothesis, would also have to account for the idiosyncratic, non-dose-related occurrence of NMS-like episodes in patients treated with drugs directly affecting dopamine; it could be used to identify other metabolic, neuromuscular, or neurotransmitter-related factors necessary to trigger a hyperthermic response.

Although hyperthermia is not typical of lithium toxicity, lithium in combination with neuroleptics has clearly been associated with the development of NMS. Lithium, which has been shown to inhibit the development of behavioral supersensitivity following neuroleptic administration, also has serotonergic properties and is increasingly recognized as having significant effects on second messenger systems. Whether these or other pharmacologic effects of lithium act in synergy with neuroleptics to enhance the toxicity of either agent remains an intriguing area of research.

A number of sympathomimetic and psychedelic drugs, in cases of overdose, have also been associated with hyperthermia. While behavioral neurotoxicity resulting in hyperactivity, agitation, or convulsions is typical of these agents and appears to account for heat production, NMS-like cases with rigidity and rhabdomyolysis have also been reported. The pharmacologic profiles of drugs in these classes leads to speculation that augmentation of dopamine, serotonin, or norepinephrine activity could be involved, although data to support this are contradictory and inconclusive. Nevertheless, hyperthermic reactions to sympathomimetic and psychedelic drugs may be particularly relevant in understanding the pathogenesis of lethal catatonia arising during the course of major psychoses.

Antidepressants, both TCAs and MAOIs, taken in overdose or used in drug combinations, have been associated with the development of hyperthermia. Some of these cases show characteristic features of NMS, including response to dantrolene. Data from animal studies provide convincing evidence that serotonergic mechanisms may be important in the development of these reactions.

In contrast, anticholinergic drugs facilitate the development of hyperthermia due to peripheral inhibition of heat loss mechanisms, but are unlikely to produce typical NMS symptoms when administered alone.

From a pathophysiologic point of view, psychoactive drug–induced hypermetabolic states may develop as a result of a disturbance in the central activity of individual monoamines, or in the interactions or balance between neurotransmitters. Apart from strong clinical evidence implicating reduced dopamine activity in NMS, clinical and animal studies of the hyperthermic effects of antidepressants, fenfluramine, and LSD implicate serotonin in the development of hyperthermia. As a number of investigators have speculated, the ratio of activity in serotonin and dopamine systems, or the mutual neuromodulatory interactions between these neurotransmitters, may serve as a unifying concept in the understanding of convergent mechanisms underlying hyperthermic drug reactions.

Contrasting effects of drugs on central neurotransmitter systems notwithstanding, NMS-like instances of drug toxicity have in common the activation of thermoregulatory effector mechanisms involved in the generation of heat by skeletal muscle. These mechanisms may represent a nonspecific final common pathway in the development of hyperthermia due to a variety of drugs, and may be mediated indirectly through neuromuscular innervation and hormonal effects, or by direct drug effects on skeletal muscle.

Chapter 4
Malignant Hyperthermia

Chapter 4

Malignant Hyperthermia

Malignant hyperthermia (MH) is an uncommon syndrome recognized as a major cause of anesthetic-related mortality among physically uncompromised patients. MH is characterized by the development of striking temperature elevation, muscle rigidity, myonecrosis, and increased oxygen consumption in susceptible patients exposed to volatile inhalational anesthetics and succinylcholine. It was first described formally by Denborough and Lovell in 1960. They reported the case of a young man who developed MH during surgery and who had a strong family history of anesthetic-related deaths. Subsequently, numerous cases were reported, and MH became the subject of several comprehensive reviews and intensive research (Ellis and Heffron 1985; Gronert 1980b; Nelson and Flewellen 1983; Rosenberg and Fletcher 1987).

While MH was attracting clinical interest, a related phenomenon in veterinary medicine was separately generating attention. It had been noted in certain breeds of pigs that the stress related to slaughter led to accelerated metabolism and degeneration of muscle, resulting in "pale, soft exudative" pork that was unsuitable for marketing. In these pigs, any stress (e.g., separation, fighting, slaughter) could result in the "porcine stress syndrome," which is characterized by increased basal metabolism, muscle rigidity, acidosis, hyperthermia, and death. A report by Hall et al. (1966) of a syndrome identical to human MH, induced in susceptible pigs exposed to halothane and succinylcholine, confirmed the porcine stress syndrome as an ideal model for investigating the pathophysiology of human MH.

The syndrome of MH is a fascinating disorder that is of interest in psychiatry and medicine as well as anesthesiology. As a hypermetabolic syndrome, MH shares many clinical features with neuroleptic malignant syndrome (NMS). Hence, consideration of the differential diagnosis between MH and NMS is of therapeutic importance in clinical settings where both anesthetics and neuroleptics are administered. Since information on MH is limited and often incomplete outside of the anesthesiology literature, it is important to review the clinical aspects of MH critically and to compare these findings to NMS. Furthermore, examination of current data on the pathophysiology of MH may provide additional insight concerning the pathophysiology of NMS and the relationship between these two disorders.

The Clinical Syndrome of Malignant Hyperthermia

Epidemiology

MH is relatively rare. Estimates of the incidence of MH vary between 1 in 15,000 to 1 in 200,000 anesthetic administrations (Nelson and Flewellen 1983; Ording 1985; Rosenberg and Fletcher 1987). It is difficult to determine the true incidence of MH susceptibility in the general population since susceptible individuals do not always develop an MH episode when exposed to anesthesia (Gronert 1980b; Halsall et al. 1979; Nelson and Flewellen 1983; Rosenberg and Fletcher 1987). Furthermore, incidence figures may vary depending on diagnostic criteria. For example, a recent study of a pediatric population in which the criterion for potential MH was the paradoxical development of masseter muscle rigidity in response to succinylcholine suggested that the incidence of MH was closer to 1 in 100 or 200 (Schwartz et al. 1984). Fifty percent or more of patients exhibiting masseter muscle spasm prove to have true MH susceptibility on further diagnostic testing, so that jaw hypertonicity may indeed by a valid, early presumptive sign of MH (Fletcher and Rosenberg 1985; Ording 1985; Rosenberg and Fletcher 1986; Rosenberg and Reed 1983). Furthermore, because of increasing knowledge of MH among anesthesiologists, anesthesia is more likely to be terminated early in suspected cases, thereby reducing the number of cases that progress to the fulminant form and reducing estimates of the incidence of the disorder.

Ording (1985) reported results of a comprehensive survey of anesthetic practices and suspected MH cases in Denmark between 1978 and 1984. Specific criteria were used to define fulminant MH episodes and suspected or abortive forms. The results showed the incidence of fulminant MH to be 1 in 250,000 general anesthetics. Fulminant MH was reported in 1 in 62,000 anesthetics in which both a potent inhalational agent and succinylcholine were administered. However, with these agents, masseter spasms occurred in 1 of 12,000 anesthetics, and other abortive forms of MH were suspected in 1 of 4,200 anesthetics. Overall, the suspicion of MH, regardless of agents used, was raised in 1 of 16,000 anesthetics.

Other demographic data indicate that MH is more common among the young. The mean age of 154 cases of suspected MH reported by Ording (1985) was 15 years (range, 0.5 to 72 years). Two-thirds of reported MH cases are between 3 and 30 years old (McPherson and Taylor 1982). Analysis by sex reveals a male predominance of roughly 2 to 1.

Genetics

A genetic predisposition to MH was noted early in the investigation of this disorder (Gronert 1980b; McPherson and Taylor 1982). Originally, MH susceptibility in humans and swine was thought to be associated with an autosomal dominant trait, possibly with reduced penetrance and variable expressivity. However, further studies have failed to reveal a consistent pattern of inheritance. Instead, polygenic and multifactorial inheritance patterns have been proposed (Gronert 1980b; Lutsky et al. 1982; Nelson and Flewellen 1983). Only about one-third of patients with MH actually report a positive family history, although 80 percent of families that have been studied diagnostically after an episode of MH contain susceptible relatives. In a review of the literature of 93 families investigated after an index episode, McPherson and Taylor (1982) found 38 percent with clearly autosomal dominant inheritance, 14 percent possibly autosomal dominant, 17 percent possibly recessive, 3 percent with other dominant myopathies, 7 percent with insufficient data, and 17 percent with isolated, sporadic cases. They suggested that MH may be conceptualized as a nonspecific syndrome that may be caused by a variety of genetic and environmental factors. A more precise understanding of the genetics of MH may depend on the development of specific and noninvasive diagnostic measures that could be used to screen for susceptibility within families.

A curious and characteristic feature of MH that confounds analyses of genetic influences is the variability of clinical expression and susceptibility for a given individual. About one-third of patients with MH report a prior history of uncomplicated anesthesia, sometimes on multiple occasions (Halsall et al. 1979; McPherson and Taylor 1982; Rosenberg and Fletcher 1987). Susceptibility may vary with age or may be modified by concurrent drug therapy, trauma, exercise, or psychological stress. The determining factors in the triggering of a specific episode in a susceptible individual are not completely understood.

Triggering Drugs and Related Factors

MH episodes are most commonly observed when volatile inhalational anesthetics such as halothane are used in combination with succinylcholine, a depolarizing skeletal muscle relaxant (Gronert 1980b; Ording 1985). Regional and intravenous anesthetics are generally considered to be safe

(Ording 1985; Paasuke and Brownell 1986a). Nitrous oxide and D-tubocurarine have been implicated as potentially weak triggering agents in a few controversial MH cases, but nitrous oxide has been safely used as a basic anesthetic for many MH-susceptible patients, and D-tubocurarine may even block the triggering effects of succinylcholine but not halothane (Gronert 1980b; Rosenberg and Fletcher 1987). Pancuronium may be the drug of choice for myoneural blockade in MH-susceptible patients, although other neuromuscular-blocking agents appear to be safe as well (Ording and Nielsen 1986; Rosenberg and Fletcher 1987).

Since succinylcholine is a known triggering agent and is also used during electroconvulsive therapy, psychiatrists should be aware of the clinical signs of MH and explore personal and family histories in relation to previous adverse reactions to anesthesia in patients evaluated for this procedure (Franks et al. 1982; Yacoub and Morrow 1986). However, MH is unlikely to occur during electroconvulsive therapy because exposure to succinylcholine is brief, inhalational agents are absent, and barbiturates may suppress reactivity (Gronert and Milde 1981; Rosenberg and Fletcher 1987). There have been no reports of MH despite the widespread use of this procedure (Sonnenklar and Rendell-Baker 1972).

Reference is often made to psychotropic drugs (e.g., antidepressants and neuroleptics), which produce reactions remarkably similar to MH. MH-susceptible patients are sometimes advised to avoid these drugs, although there is no evidence that MH susceptibility correlates with hyperthermic reactions to these agents. There are no reported cases of NMS reactions in MH-susceptible patients treated with neuroleptics. On the contrary, neuroleptics have been used to treat MH episodes (Kolb et al. 1982) and appear to delay the onset and attenuate the severity of the syndrome in MH-susceptible swine when administered prior to halothane (Somers and McLoughlin 1982). Similarly, tricyclic antidepressants have been administered to MH-susceptible patients without adverse effects (Richter and Joffe 1987).

The report of one patient with biopsy-proven MH susceptibility, who died from a typical MH-like reaction associated with cocaine and alcohol, suggests that stimulants may trigger MH (Loghmanee and Tobak 1986) (see Chapter 3). In addition, hyperthermic reactions to phencyclidine may be related to MH since ketamine, a similar arylcyclohexylamine anesthetic, has triggered MH episodes in patients with known MH susceptibility (Page et al. 1972; Roervik and Stovner 1974; Rosenberg and Fletcher 1987).

Apart from effects of anesthesia, hypermetabolic responses in swine can be elicited by exposure to exercise, heat stress, anoxia, apprehension, or excitement (Chambers and Hall 1987; D'Allaire and DeRoth 1986; Gronert 1980; Ording et al. 1985). These features of the porcine stress syndrome have suggested that central or sympathetic nervous system mechanisms may facilitate the development of acute MH episodes (Rosenberg and Fletcher 1987).

In humans, the influence of nonanesthetic or stress-related factors is less clear. Smith et al. (1986) found significant correlations between state anxiety, hormonal secretion, and MH susceptibility as demonstrated by diagnostic biopsy. Conflicting results have been obtained from studies of the response of patients with MH to exercise and heat. Campbell et al. (1981) initially found hormonal and biochemical abnormalities in subjects with MH compared to controls in response to food and mild exercise. Subsequently, the same group (Campbell et al. 1983) found a rise of core temperature greater than controls in MH-susceptible subjects exposed to severe exercise, which they attributed to impaired heat dissipation resulting from inhibition of vasodilation. This, in combination with elevated serum-free fatty acids, suggested that an abnormality of sympathetic activity existed in subjects with MH. Green et al. (1987) recently reported no differences between subjects with MH and controls in response to long-term, moderate exercise when demands are placed primarily on aerobic metabolism. In addition, other investigators have been unable to find differences between subjects with MH and controls exposed to exercise (Ayling et al. 1986; Rutberg et al. 1986).

There have been a few reports of "awake" episodes of MH, unrelated to anesthesia, which were associated with stress, positive diagnostic tests, and response to dantrolene (Gronert et al. 1980; Kelemen et al. 1986), although these remain controversial. Other investigators have suggested that patients with MH are stress sensitive, may develop a variety of "awake" symptoms, and are prone to sudden death (Ranklev et al. 1985; Wingard and Gatz 1978). Along these lines, Meyers and Meyers (1982) proposed that MH and NMS were manifestations of a "thermic stress syndrome" in humans, which could be triggered by a variety of mechanisms and which also encompassed heatstroke, sudden death in athletes, and other conditions. While these disorders may eventuate in a similar clinical picture of hypermetabolism and extreme hyperthermia, etiologic mechanisms appear quite different; there is scant evidence at this time to suggest a common, genetic vulnerability among patients with these disorders (Clark and Lipton 1984).

Nevertheless, reports of stress-related or "awake" episodes of MH are intriguing from a psychiatric viewpoint as they suggest that MH may be the anesthetic-induced manifestation of a generalized human stress syndrome analogous to the porcine model. Further understanding of these cases and their relationship to MH during anesthesia may shed light on mechanisms underlying psychophysiologic reactions to stress in humans, including lethal catatonia and sudden death in psychiatric patients (see Chapter 5). They may also help elucidate the role of stress in the development of NMS episodes.

Clinical Manifestations of MH

Once MH is triggered during anesthesia, a fulminant

hypermetabolic response ensues in which body temperature may increase 1 °C every 5 minutes. Elevated temperatures are invariably present within the first 1 to 2 hours of induction. However, several recent reports suggest that MH-like episodes may be more insidious, occurring up to several hours postoperatively (Grinberg et al. 1983; Souliere et al. 1986).

The first major chemical change reflecting increased aerobic and anaerobic metabolism during MH is the production of acidosis accompanied by a drop in blood pH and a rise in blood PCO_2. Metabolic acidosis is primarily due to lactic acid production. Thus a rise in blood PCO_2, which can be monitored during anesthesia, may be one of the earliest signs of MH, preceding a rise in temperature by several minutes (Dunn et al. 1985; Neubauer and Kaufman 1985).

Early clinical signs of MH include unexplained tachycardia or change in blood pressure. Another sign that may herald the onset of MH is paradoxical trismus or masseter muscle rigidity after halothane induction and succinylcholine administration (Badgwell and Heavner 1984; Gronert 1980b; Ording 1985; Rosenberg and Fletcher 1986). MH in its full-blown form is further characterized by signs of circulatory and hypermetabolic stress. Circulating catecholamines are strikingly elevated.

Virtually all pigs and approximately 75 percent of humans developing MH show muscle rigidity (Gronert 1980b). The rigidity and hypermetabolism of MH results in increased membrane permeability with release into serum of muscle enzymes, myoglobin, and ions. Subsequently, the patient may experience arrhythmias, cardiac arrest, cardiovascular collapse, disseminated intravascular coagulation, or renal failure. The mortality of MH was originally estimated to be 60 to 70 percent, but with increased recognition, early cessation of anesthesia, and treatment with dantrolene more recent estimates of mortality range from 10 to 30 percent (Gronert 1980b; Ording 1985). Among survivors of fulminant

MH episodes, some may be left with evidence of diffuse brain damage (Mazzia and Simon 1978).

Treatment of MH

Therapy rests on the early recognition of signs of MH and termination of anesthetic administration. In mild cases recognized early this may suffice to abort an episode. However, more fulminant episodes require intensive physiologic monitoring and urgent therapeutic interventions to maintain metabolic and cardiovascular status and to lower body temperature during the episode and for 24 to 48 hours after recovery.

Dantrolene sodium, or l-([5-(p-nitrophenyl)-furfurylidene] amino) hydantoin sodium hydrate, is the recommended treatment for MH, but in order to reverse the condition it must be administered promptly while muscle perfusion is still adequate (Gronert 1980b; Kolb et al. 1982). Dantrolene was initially developed as an antispasmodic agent because of its unique properties as a peripheral skeletal muscle relaxant. Its efficacy appears to depend on actions outside the central nervous system. Dantrolene has been shown to have no effect on electrical properties of muscle or on neuromuscular transmission (Colton and Colton 1979; Ellis and Bryant 1972; Ellis and Carpenter 1972). Further studies have shown that dantrolene interferes with the excitation-contraction process in skeletal muscle; its site of action is at a step subsequent to membrane depolarization. It has been shown that dantrolene diminishes the twitch tension and contracture response of skeletal muscle to diverse agents by affecting calcium movement inside the muscle fiber, resulting in a reduction of free intracellular calcium concentrations (Lopez et al. 1987). There are conflicting data, however, as to whether this occurs due to inhibition of influx of trigger calcium from the sarcolemma or transverse tubules (Halsall and Ellis 1983; Putney and Bianchi 1974), or is due to attenuation of calcium release from sarcoplasmic reticulum or other intracellular stores (Colton and Colton 1979; Ellis and Carpenter 1974; Gronert 1980).

Regardless of the mechanism of action, it was noted that dantrolene was effective in inhibiting halothane- and caffeine-induced contractures in muscle from MH-susceptible swine (Anderson et al. 1978; Kerr et al. 1978; Nelson and Denborough 1977; Nelson and Flewellen 1979). Dantrolene was also found to be effective in the treatment of MH episodes in the intact pig (Gronert 1980b; Harrison 1975). Subsequently, a number of case reports confirmed the efficacy of dantrolene in treating human MH.

Kolb et al. (1982), in a multicenter trial, found that intravenous dantrolene at a mean dose of 2.5 mg/kg produced a significant decrement in signs of hypermetabolism in 11 patients with definite or probable MH. They also found that administration of dantrolene more than 24 hours after the diagnosis of MH failed to prevent mortality. While this was an open, nonrandomized study without controls, the infrequent and ordinarily catastrophic nature of MH enhances the clinical significance of these data (Forrest 1982).

During an MH episode, dantrolene appears to dampen metabolic activity and diminish the associated acidosis, ion fluxes, and sympathetic stimulation more predictably than symptomatic treatment. The recommended intravenous dose is 2.5 mg/kg, which may be repeated every 5 to 10 minutes to a total dose of 10 mg/kg (Ellis and Heffron 1985; Gronert 1980b; Rosenberg and Fletcher 1987). Dantrolene should probably be continued for 24 to 48 hours after control is achieved in order to prevent symptom recurrence, although standard guidelines for this have not been developed (Ellis and Halsall 1980; Gronert 1980b; Rosenberg and Fletcher 1987). Preoperative preparation with dantrolene sodium (2.5 mg/kg over 30 minutes intravenously) has also been recommended for known MH-susceptible patients (Ellis and Heffron 1985; Rosenberg and Fletcher 1987). Dantrolene has been associated with muscle weakness as a side effect

(Oikkonen et al. 1987; Rosenberg and Fletcher 1987). Although hepatic dysfunction has been reported with long-term oral dantrolene administration, serious toxicity has not been reported with doses effective in treating MH (Gronert 1980b; Kolb et al. 1982).

Diagnosis of MH Susceptibility

Apart from management of the acute episode perioperatively, the treatment of MH can be greatly enhanced by preventive measures based on reliable identification of susceptible patients preoperatively. Evaluation of susceptibility includes a careful history and physical examination, focusing on anesthetic exposures and evidence of neuromuscular disease (Ellis and Heffron 1985; Larach et al. 1987). A family history concerning surgical procedures and specific anesthetic agents is crucial.

Elevation of serum creatine phosphokinase (CPK) was thought to be useful as a basic screening test, with abnormal results obtained in up to 70 percent of susceptible patients. However, a recent study by Paasuke and Brownell (1986b) suggested that while CPK may correlate with MH susceptibility in some families, it is generally insensitive and nonspecific as a measure of susceptibility and correlates poorly with in vitro muscle contracture studies. They suggested that an elevation of CPK obligates the clinician to search for other possible causes of this finding.

A variety of other diagnostic tests and biologic markers have been proposed, including erythrocyte osmotic fragility, nuclear magnetic resonance, platelet adenosine triphosphate (ATP) depletion in response to halothane, abnormal platelet aggregation, electrodiagnostic tests, abnormal muscle enzymes, and calcium uptake, but none of these have been confirmed as reliable (Ellis and Heffron 1985; Olgin et al. 1988; Ording 1988; Paasuke and Brownell 1986b; Rosenberg and Fletcher 1987).

As a result, the most extensively studied and generally accepted screening test for MH susceptibility remains the in vitro skeletal muscle contracture test. Patients with abortive or suggestive episodes of MH, as well as relatives of patients with documented MH episodes or MH susceptibility, are potential candidates for diagnostic muscle biopsy (Rosenberg and Reed 1983). The test is based on the original observation by Kalow et al. (1970) that muscle from susceptible patients has a lower contracture threshold to caffeine in vitro. Subsequently the test was refined and expanded in several laboratories around the world when it was found that exposure to other agents—including halothane, potassium, and succinylcholine—revealed heightened sensitivity or decreased threshold for contracture in susceptible muscle. The main problems with this test are its invasive nature, the lack of standardization of procedures and diagnostic criteria between laboratories, and the limited availability of control data. Nevertheless, it has been considered up to 90 percent reliable in the evaluation of MH susceptibility (Gronert 1980b).

Recently, there have been a number of attempts to standardize procedures and diagnostic criteria between laboratories (The European Malignant Hyperpyrexia Group 1984; Rosenberg and Reed 1983). Additional studies have focused on assessment of the sensitivity and specificity of the test. For example, the contracture response of swine muscle to test drugs has been shown to correlate with documented MH reactions, and reliable dose-response data are available to support the test in this animal model (McGrath et al. 1984; Nelson et al. 1975; Okumura 1979).

Similarly, studies in muscle from MH-susceptible patients and normal controls have generally supported the sensitivity and specificity of the halothane-caffeine contracture test. Although use of a battery of test drugs is still recommended, the responses to halothane and caffeine appear to be sensitive and specific measures of MH susceptibility. Rosenberg and Reed (1983), using halothane (1 percent), correctly classified 15 normal controls and six patients with documented MH reactions. Larach et al. (1987) reported a significant association between the presence of two or more adverse reactions during anesthesia and MH susceptibility as determined by testing with halothane (2 to 3 percent) or caffeine (2 mM). Ording et al. (1984) could distinguish 31 controls from nine patients with MH on the basis of the contracture response to 0.5 to 2 percent halothane and 0.5 to 2 mM caffeine. They also found that halothane was the most sensitive test; 88 percent of positive patients had an abnormal response to this drug. In a further study by the same group (Ranklev et al. 1986), no specimens from 12 healthy subjects showed a contracture response to 2 percent or less halothane, or 2 mM or less caffeine, thereby supporting the criteria established by the European Malignant Hyperpyrexia Group (1984). Using the same criteria, Ording and Skovgaard (1987) reported that none of 20 normal controls were MH susceptible whereas one patient with classic fulminant MH tested positive. In earlier studies, Nelson et al. (1977) studied the response to halothane in muscle from 57 normal subjects and found that 18 showed contractures greater than 0.1 g, and four of these showed responses greater than 0.5 g at halothane concentrations of 0.4 to 4 percent. Nonetheless, they recommended halothane as a sensitive means of testing susceptibility but advised exposure to other test drugs to enhance the reliability of the procedure. Moulds and Denborough (1974) studied contractures in normal muscle and found small, slow contractures in response to halothane in only two of 18 muscle strips tested. Finally, Gronert (1980a) reported no contractures following halothane (2 percent) administration in muscle obtained from 33 patients with normal muscle function. False-negative contracture tests, resulting in subsequent MH episodes during anesthesia, have not been reported (Ellis and Halsall 1986).

Although data on specificity of the contracture test in regard to normal controls are increasing, specificity of positive test results for true MH susceptibility in patients with underlying neuromuscular disorders remains controversial (Ellis and Heffron 1985; Gronert 1983; Rosenberg and Fletcher 1987). For example, positive test results have been reported in patients with central core disease, muscular dystrophy, and myotonia congenita, and in parents of children with sudden infant death (Ellis and Heffron 1985; Ording et al. 1984; Paasuke and Brownell 1986b; Rosenberg and Fletcher 1987). Whether these results represent true MH susceptibility or merely reflect underlying muscle pathology unrelated to MH is unclear. In some of these cases, positive findings have correlated with clinical MH episodes. At the very least, the finding of abnormal contracture test results indicative of MH susceptibility in these disorders further supports the conceptualization of MH as a syndrome rather than a specific disease.

Pathogenesis

Effects on the central nervous system in MH appear to be secondary to elevated temperature, acidosis, hyperkalemia, and hypoxia (Gronert 1980b; Gronert et al. 1988). Some data, however, suggest more fundamental neural involvement. For example, histologic examination of muscle from patients with MH has revealed signs of neurogenic as well as myogenic changes (Harriman 1988; Heiman-Patterson et al., unpublished data). Based on motor unit counting, Britt et al. (1977) suggested that MH involves motor neurons as well as muscle, although this approach was criticized by Gronert (1980b). Ahern (1985) reported that electrical stimulation of the lumbosacral and brachial plexes resulted in a prolonged increase in metabolism and catecholamine levels in MH-susceptible pigs, not unlike the increase observed in response to halothane or succinylcholine. However, contrary evidence, such as lack of rigidity in a limb isolated by a tourniquet during episodes of rigid MH, argue against neural initiation of MH (Gronert 1980b).

In relation to the association between MH and NMS, Mereu et al. (1984) reported that general anesthesia with chloral hydrate, pentobarbital, or halothane in rats paralyzed with succinylcholine significantly increased the firing rate of dopaminergic neurons in the substantia nigra. Furthermore, pretreatment with anesthetics inhibited the effect of haloperidol and sulpiride in stimulating the firing rate and activating tyrosine hydroxylase. The authors suggested that excitation of dopaminergic neurons produced by neuroleptics and anesthetics may be mediated by the same neuronal mechanisms. Further investigation of this effect may be warranted, especially if it can be shown that the compensatory increase in dopamine synthesis in response to postsynaptic blockade by neuroleptics has some role in the development of hyperthermia during NMS (see Chapter 3).

Correlations between central dopamine activity and MH susceptibility have also been proposed by Draper et al. (1984). These investigators found that dopamine concentrations in the caudate nucleus of stress-susceptible pigs were significantly lower than in stress-resistant pigs, whereas epinephrine and norepinephrine concentrations were similar in both groups.

Relatively greater interest as well as controversy concerns the finding of abnormal sympathetic responses in MH and whether they contribute to the initiation of MH episodes (Gronert 1980b). There are several reasons to suspect autonomic involvement in human and porcine MH (Williams 1976). In pigs, and perhaps in humans, MH may develop in response to stress. Heat and exercise have been associated with physiologic changes in pigs and humans, and have resulted in MH episodes in susceptible pigs (Campbell et al. 1981, 1983; D'Allaire and DeRoth 1986; Ording et al. 1985). However, other investigators found no differences between patients with MH and controls in the response of temperature, metabolic rate, and catecholamines to exercise (Ayling et al. 1986; Green et al. 1987; Rutberg et al. 1986).

Signs of sympathetic stimulation and elevated catecholamines are observed clinically during MH. In some studies, sympathetic (alpha-adrenergic) agonists triggered MH episodes, and catecholamine depletion in some animals abolished halothane sensitivity (Lucke et al. 1979). Furthermore, exposure to cocaine, a sympathomimetic agent, has resulted in MH and death in one patient with known MH susceptibility (Loghmanee and Tobak 1986).

Gronert (1980b) speculated that the effects of alpha-agonists were mediated indirectly through increased peripheral vasoconstriction, which would result in tissue hypoxia and heat generation leading to a generalized MH reaction. Gronert et al. (1977, 1980b) demonstrated that sympathetic agonists had no direct effect on metabolism in isolated muscle specimens obtained from stress-susceptible pigs and that inhibition of sympathetic activity by spinal anesthesia failed to prevent the occurrence of MH in swine. Recently, Gronert et al. (1986) demonstrated that sympathetic stimulation related to hypercarbia did not stimulate abnormal metabolism in muscle from susceptible pigs. Gronert (1980) suggested that initiation of stress responses in intact swine is related to somatic motor and sympathetic stimulation of abnormal skeletal muscle, and not to a disorder of the somatic or sympathetic nervous system.

Thus the evidence for a primary neural etiology for MH remains unconvincing. However, a facilitory role for catecho-Allamines and the sympathetic nervous system in the development of MH episodes merits further study because (1) membrane abnormalities in MH may not be limited to muscle tissue (Denborough 1978; Gronert 1980b; Klip et al. 1986; Mickelson et al. 1987); (2) epinephrine enhances neuromuscular transmission, glycogenolysis, and muscle tone through intracellular changes in free calcium ions (Bowman and Nott 1969; Gallant et al. 1980); and (3) sympathomimetics (e.g., amphetamine and cocaine) have been reported in association with MH-like hyperthermic reactions (see Chapter 3).

Overall, clinical and laboratory evidence favors the hypothesis that MH is of primary myogenic origin (Gronert et al. 1988). Some families have obvious skeletal muscle abnormalities, and conversely, patients with disorders of muscle (e.g., muscular dystrophy) may be at risk for MH (Gronert 1980b). In addition, serum CPK values may be elevated at rest in up to 70 percent of affected patients and in most swine, suggesting that basal metabolic processes in MH muscle may be increased compared to normal. Similarly, the earliest changes in MH appear in the venous effluent from skeletal muscle as decreases in pH or PO_2 and increases in lactate, potassium, or temperature (Gronert 1980b), reflecting increased muscle metabolism. These changes have been shown to precede increases in body temperature, heart rate, catecholamines, and muscle tone.

Although histologic examination of porcine and human muscle has failed to reveal a specific pathologic pattern, muscle contracture studies have confirmed the presence of abnormal functional responses in muscle from affected individuals. Halothane and caffeine contractures in susceptible muscle appear to be mediated by postjunctional mechanisms related to excitation-contraction coupling. Also, dantrolene is effective in MH, probably based on its actions in inhibiting calcium release in muscle cells (Gronert 1980b; Lopez et al. 1987; Nelson and Denborough 1977; Rosenberg 1979).

Investigations measuring electromechanical coupling time (Nelson et al. 1983) and high-energy phosphates by nuclear magnetic resonance (Cozzone et al. 1985; Ellis and Heffron 1985; Olgin et al. 1988) or other methods (Hall and Lucke 1983) provide further evidence of hypermetabolism in MH resulting from an alteration in the excitation-contraction coupling mechanism. These changes could be effected by an abnormal elevation of intracellular calcium. Nelson and Chausmer (1981) originally reported lower concentrations of calcium in muscle from MH-susceptible pigs and suggested that the muscle defect in MH is associated with a calcium storage pool in equilibrium with extracellular calcium. However, Nelson et al. (1987a) later found no difference in calcium content, although magnesium content was greater, in muscle obtained from patients with MH compared to controls. More recently, Lopez et al. (1985, 1987) used selective microelectrodes to demonstrate significantly higher resting myoplasmic-free calcium concentrations, which could be reduced by dantrolene, in patients with MH compared to controls.

A rise in calcium could explain the muscle rigidity, acidosis, and hyperthermia found in MH. Elevation of myoplasmic calcium could cause further calcium release from intracellular stores or from the extracellular space. These calcium ions would combine with troponin, activate myosin ATPase, and stimulate actin-myosin interactions, resulting in the hydrolysis of ATP to adenosine diphosphate (ADP) and phosphate and the production of heat and muscle contraction. Calcium also activates phosphorylase-mediated effects on glycogen, resulting in production of lactic acid, carbon dioxide, and heat. Finally, elevated calcium concentrations may uncouple oxidative phosphorylation, thereby decreasing ATP production and further accelerating oxygen consumption and the production of lactic acid, carbon dioxide, and heat (Britt 1979; Denborough 1986).

Under normal conditions, depolarization of the muscle membrane at the myoneural junction is propagated through the transverse tubular (T-tubule) system. This signal is then transmitted by mechanisms that remain unclear to the terminal cisternae of the sarcoplasmic reticulum, which releases calcium to initiate contractile processes, and removes calcium from the myoplasm to terminate contraction. The exact site of the defect in MH resulting in a rise of myoplasmic calcium is unknown (Ellis and Heffron 1985; Gronert 1980b). While a number of investigators have identified abnormalities of calcium transport in mitochondria (Gallant et al. 1986; Heffron 1986), current evidence suggests that impaired uptake or augmented release of calcium from sarcoplasmic reticulum (Condrescu et al. 1987; Mickelson et al. 1986; Nelson et al. 1986, 1987b; O'Brien 1986a, 1986b; Ohnishi et al. 1986; Takagi and Araki 1986) and defective calcium transport across the sarcolemma (Gallant et al. 1986; Heffron 1986; Klip et al. 1986; Mickelson et al. 1987; Rock and Kozak-Reiss 1987) in response to depolarization, calcium-induced calcium release, or pharmacologic triggering agents represent the most likely defects in MH.

While a hypersensitive calcium-release mechanism of sarcoplasmic reticulum and/or abnormal sarcolemmal calcium transport are emerging as the possible defects underlying MH, a number of investigators have begun to explore biochemical alterations that would account for these defects. For example, structural abnormalities of muscle cell and organelle membranes have been proposed (Marjanen et al. 1984; Ohnishi et al. 1986; Oku et al. 1983). Intracellular second messenger systems, such as those involving cyclic adenosine monophosphate (AMP), may be abnormal in MH-susceptible subjects (Stanec and Stefano 1984).

In addition, there may be some involvement of the intracellular calcium messenger system associated with phosphoinositide metabolism (Rasmussen 1986a, 1986b). It has been reported that inositol triphosphate, resulting from hydrolysis of phosphatidylinositol in the plasma membrane, acts as a chemical second messenger between transverse tubular membrane depolarization and the calcium-release process at the sarcoplasmic reticulum in skeletal muscle (Vergara et al. 1985). In addition, inositol triphosphate-induced calcium release may be antagonized by dantrolene (Kojima et al. 1984). Further examination of phospholipid metabolism as a chemical intermediary pathway between T-tubule depolarization and calcium release from sarcoplasmic reticulum may shed additional light on mechanisms underlying changes in calcium transport in MH. In fact, several investigators have speculated that the biochemical defect in MH may be associated with abnormal phospholipid metabolism, specifically elevation of phospholipase A_2 activity, which may result in altered membrane permeability and elevated sarcoplasmic calcium (Cheah and Cheah 1985; Fletcher et al. 1986).

Comparison with NMS

As NMS gained recognition, several investigators noted the clinical similarities to MH and suggested that these syndromes may share a common pathophysiology (Bourgeois et al. 1971; Meltzer 1973; Itoh et al. 1977). However, there are important differences between MH and NMS. While the incidence of MH has been estimated at 1 in 15,000 to 1 in 200,000 (Ording 1985), the incidence of NMS may be between 1 in 100 to 1 in 5,000 (Caroff and Mann 1988). Incidence rates for both conditions vary considerably depending on diagnostic criteria. MH and NMS are both more commonly reported among males by a factor of 2 to 1. While MH may occur at any age, the mean age has been reported as 15 years (Ording 1985), whereas the mean age of reported NMS cases is approximately 38 years (Klein et al. 1985; Levenson 1985). While both conditions may be more common in the young, the older mean age in NMS reports may reflect the fact that young children are less likely to be exposed to neuroleptics than to anesthetics. In contrast to reports of variable genetic patterns in families with MH, including sporadic cases, there have been no reports of familial susceptibility to NMS.

Pharmacologic differences between MH and NMS are underscored by the fact that sensitivity to neuroleptics has not been reported in MH-susceptible patients. In fact, droperidol has been considered a safe anesthetic agent for patients with MH (Kolb et al. 1982; Rosenberg and Fletcher 1987), although this neuroleptic has been associated with NMS episodes (Bernstein and Scherokman 1986; Bourgeois et al. 1981; Krivosic-Horber et al. 1987; Lagarde et al. 1986; Patel and Bristow 1987; Parini et al. 1984; Reis et al. 1983). Moreover, neuroleptics have been reported to delay and attenuate MH episodes in swine exposed to halothane

(Somers and McLoughlin 1982). Conversely, episodes of MH have not been reported in patients with NMS during anesthesia.

While stress, exercise, and heat may precipitate the porcine stress syndrome, the role of such factors in triggering MH episodes is uncertain. Elevated catecholamines and sympathetic activation may facilitate the development of MH. Catecholamines are also markedly elevated in NMS. Recently, Shalev et al. (1988) proposed that heat stress may facilitate the development of NMS. One of the most puzzling characteristics of both syndromes is the fact that triggering drugs appear to be necessary but not sufficient to precipitate hyperthermic episodes. Patients who develop MH or NMS show variability in clinical expression of the disorder such that repeated episodes may not be apparent during previous or subsequent exposures to the same drugs. Other as yet unidentified stress or risk factors are apparently involved in the development of both disorders.

While MH usually develops rapidly during induction of anesthesia, NMS develops less precipitously. However, delayed onset or recrudescence of MH has been reported, and may pose a diagnostic dilemma in patients also receiving neuroleptics during the postoperative recovery period. The differences between MH and NMS in rapidity of onset may in part reflect differences in the pharmacokinetics and routes of administration of the respective triggering drugs, or may reflect basic differences in etiology, that is, myogenic versus neurogenic mechanisms (Ellis and Heffron 1985).

MH and NMS both present clinically as hypermetabolic syndromes, usually with pronounced muscle rigidity, rhabdomyolysis, and hyperthermia. Clark and Lipton (1984) suggested that unlike MH, temperatures during NMS uncommonly exceeded 40 °C. They proposed that this difference may result from the more gradual onset of NMS, allowing for therapeutic intervention to limit hyperthermia, and the preservation of sweating in NMS compared to MH. However, in a recent review, temperatures exceeding 40 °C were present in 39 percent of NMS cases reported between 1980 and 1987 (Caroff and Mann 1988). In contrast to MH, relaxation of muscle rigidity has been achieved in some NMS cases using curare and pancuronium, suggesting that the rigidity in NMS is of neurogenic origin (Morris et al. 1980; Sangal and Dimitrijevic 1985). However, D-tubocurarine and pancuronium have also been reported to block the effects of succinylcholine and carbachol, but not halothane, in triggering MH (Gronert 1980b). Furthermore, nondepolarizing muscle relaxants may delay or attenuate the effects of halothane in swine, although a similar delay has been obtained with thiopental by unknown mechanisms (Gronert 1980). Although comparative physiologic data, especially during early stages of NMS, are not consistently reported, available data on acid-base analysis in patients with NMS reveal that metabolic acidosis is common, as in MH (Benoit et al. 1981; Boles 1982; Caroff and Mann 1988; Eles et al. 1984; Hashimoto et al. 1984; Henderson and Wooten 1981; Weinberg and Twersky 1983).

The mortality rate from MH has declined from 70 percent in the 1960s to about 10 percent in the 1980s; the mortality rate from NMS has declined from 30 percent in the 1970s to 10 percent currently with virtually no deaths in recently reported series of cases (Caroff and Mann 1988; Rosenberg and Fletcher 1987).

As reviewed in Chapter 1, dantrolene has also been used successfully in NMS cases. Although this is consistent with an association between NMS and MH, the effect of dantrolene in limiting hypermetabolic activity in skeletal muscle is nonspecific. Alterations at any level of the neuromuscular or thermoregulatory axes that result in heat generation in muscle may be compensated for by dantrolene. The nonspecificity of dantrolene is supported by its efficacy in treating hyperthermia associated with environmental heat stress (Lydiatt and Hill 1981; Paasuke 1984), L-asparaginase toxicity (Smithson et al. 1983), and antidepressant overdose

162

(Kaplan et al. 1986; Ritchie 1983; Verilli et al. 1987; Yamawaki 1986).

To date, there have been several studies that utilized the caffeine-halothane contracture test to determine whether patients with NMS would show responses consistent with MH susceptibility. Tollefson (1982), Scarlett et al. (1983), Ellis and Heffron (1985), and Merry et al. (1986) reported negative results in individual patients who recovered from NMS episodes. Krivosic-Horber et al. (1987) performed contracture testing on six survivors of NMS. Using the protocol advocated by the European Malignant Hyperthermia Group (1984), they found that five patients were not susceptible and one showed an equivocal response to caffeine. In contrast, Denborough et al. (1984), Araki et al. (1988), and Caroff et al. (1987a) reported positive test results. Caroff et al. (1987a) reported that the contracture response to halothane was consistent with MH susceptibility in five of seven patients with NMS, based on diagnostic criteria proposed in earlier studies (Rosenberg and Reed 1983). Reanalyzing the data in this study using the European criteria (European Malignant Hyperthermia Group 1984) alters the results such that only one NMS patient was MH susceptible, two were negative, and four showed equivocal responses. By these criteria, five of six controls were negative and one showed an equivocal response for MH susceptibility. Furthermore, Caroff et al. (1987a) commented that the interpretation of positive test results in patients with NMS depends on the specificity of the association between abnormal in vitro responses and MH susceptibility. In other words, positive contracture test results in NMS may represent false positives and result from coincidental changes in muscle resulting from rather than causing NMS. In fact, examination of skeletal muscle morphology in the patients reported by Caroff et al. (1987a) and Araki et al. (1988) revealed nonspecific histologic abnormalities in each patient (Heiman-Patterson et al., unpublished data).

Differences in results of contracture testing may reflect heterogeneity among patients with NMS in anesthetic sensitivity, but differences between investigators in the extent of data reported and the lack of standardization of procedures, control groups, and diagnostic criteria preclude a meaningful comparison of data across studies. Since the specificity of the contracture test requires further study, and in view of the fact that a number of patients with NMS have tolerated general anesthesia without incident (see Chapter 1), it would be premature and unwarranted to conclude that positive contracture test results signify true MH susceptibility in patients with NMS. At the same time, anesthesia should be carefully monitored in patients recovering from NMS because rhabdomyolysis and general physical debilitation may predispose them to other adverse effects (George and Wood 1987).

Investigations of the pathophysiology of MH may have relevance for research in NMS. Although clinical evidence suggests that NMS is a disorder of central nervous system function, the clinical and laboratory similarities between NMS and MH support the possibility of common mechanisms of heat generation in the two disorders (Caroff 1980, Caroff et al. 1987a). Although investigations of central and autonomic mechanisms in both conditions are worth pursuing, study of neuroleptic pharmacology on muscle may also be revealing. For example, muscle as an excitable tissue may serve as a model for neuroleptic actions on neuronal function. Moreover, muscle contractures due to direct administration of phenothiazines in vitro have been demonstrated in skeletal muscle obtained from laboratory animals. This effect appears to be mediated by an increase in myoplasmic calcium resulting from drug effects on intracellular calcium storage structures (Andersson 1972; Balzer and Hellenbrecht 1969; Collins et al. 1987; Kelkar et al. 1974; Takagi 1981). Phenothiazines induce contractures in human muscle as well, albeit at high concentrations (Caroff et al. 1983), which raises the question as to whether extrapyramidal rigidity in NMS could be further augmented by direct effects of neuroleptics on skeletal muscle.

At a biochemical level, phenothiazines have been reported to affect phosphoinositide metabolism (Walenga et al. 1981). They are potent calmodulin antagonists, may inhibit calmodulin-dependent phospholipase A_2, and may have dose-related effects on phospholipase C. These actions could potentially alter neuronal and skeletal muscle function (Vergara et al. 1985) by inducing abnormalities in the release of calcium as an intracellular second messenger (Rasmussen 1986a, 1986b).

Conclusion

MH remains a significant clinical problem and area of research with relevance for psychiatrists as well as anesthesiologists. The clinical and physiologic events associated with MH have been extensively studied. The porcine stress syndrome in pigs continues to provide a valuable animal model for this disorder. Investigations of MH have provided a scientific rationale for the development of diagnostic screening tests and improved treatment with the use of dantrolene.

Nevertheless, a number of intriguing issues remain. The factors involved in triggering an MH episode are unclear. This puzzle is underscored by the lack of consistent effects of anesthetics in triggering MH episodes in MH-susceptible individuals. The role of stress and sympathetic activity in facilitating the triggering mechanism during anesthesia or in awake episodes is controversial and unresolved. The relative influence of genetic and environmental influences is unclear. The validity, sensitivity, and specificity of the in vitro caffeine-halothane contracture test for MH susceptibility requires further examination; less invasive diagnostic tests are desirable. The significance of positive test results in patients with unrelated neuromuscular disorders remains unclear. Further data are required to determine whether a biochemical defect can be identified to account for abnormalities of intracellular calcium regulation and the resulting clinical manifestations of MH.

Many of the same questions are pertinent to a more complete understanding of mechanisms underlying NMS. Are similar factors, possibly affecting different levels of the neuromuscular, autonomic, and thermoregulatory systems simultaneously, involved in the development of NMS? What role does the sympathetic nervous system play in NMS? While impairment of central heat loss mechanisms by neuroleptics contributes to thermoregulatory dysfunction, NMS appears to be primarily a consequence of excessive heat production derived from skeletal muscle hypermetabolism. Even though substantial clinical evidence implicates inhibitory effects of neuroleptics on dopamine activity in the brain as the basis for the development of muscle rigidity and heat generation, could hypermetabolism in NMS be due in part to neuroleptic-induced dysfunction in skeletal muscle? In addition, could skeletal muscle dysfunction in predisposed individuals account for the rare and idiosyncratic occurrence of NMS among patients treated with neuroleptics?

Investigations of central mechanisms in NMS and the development of relevant animal or in vitro models should be pursued. Similarities between MH and NMS suggest that investigations of biochemical and physiological effects of neuroleptics on skeletal muscle may also be important. Although MH and NMS may be considered separate disorders with distinct pharmacologic etiologies, they appear to culminate in a similar alteration of membrane function that serves as a final common pathway affecting calcium movement and energetic processes in skeletal muscle.

Chapter 5
Lethal Catatonia

Chapter 5
Lethal Catatonia

*I*n 1934 Stauder described a fulminating psychotic disorder characterized by extreme motor excitement followed by stuporous rigidity, cardiovascular collapse, coma, and death. The entire course, passing through excitement into stupor, involved mounting hyperthermia, clouding of consciousness, and progressive autonomic dysfunction. Stauder termed the condition "lethal catatonia," although the disorder had been discussed previously by Calmeil (1832), Bell (1849), and numerous others prior to Stauder. Competing terminologies include Bell's mania, mortal catatonia, fatal catatonia, acute delirious mania, manic-depressive exhaustion death, psychotic exhaustion syndrome, hypertoxic schizophrenia, delirium acutum, delire aigu, and Scheid's cyanotic syndrome, among others. In view of the wide citation of Stauder's (1934) article, we use lethal catatonia (LC) here as a generic term for this disorder.

LC was the subject of much U.S. and foreign literature throughout the preneuroleptic era. Although the prevalence of LC may have declined worldwide, coincident with the introduction of modern psychopharmacologic agents, it has remained widely discussed. In contrast, the pertinent North American literature has been limited to a small number of single case reports, with an almost complete lack of reference to the historical literature or the contemporary foreign work.

Furthermore, many descriptions of LC from the preneuroleptic era appear quite similar and perhaps indistinguishable from contemporary descriptions of neuroleptic malignant syndrome (NMS). We were intrigued as to what relationship, if any, exists between the two disorders. Are cases currently identified as NMS actually LC of old, now mistakenly perceived as a complication of neuroleptic treatment? In attempting to address this question, we found that the dearth of information on LC in contemporary English-language publications underscores the need for a current review. As Lindesay (1986) has commented, to clarify the relationship between NMS, NMS-like syndromes, and LC, "it will first be necessary for us to rediscover lethal catatonia" (p. 342).

Clinical Presentation: Preneuroleptic Era

Alzheimer, Kraepelin, and Bleuler were among the many physicians of the preneuroleptic era to discuss LC. Despite diversity of nomenclature, there is much consistency in early clinical accounts of LC suggesting the following composite clinical sketch (Table 5.1). A prodromal phase lasting about 2 weeks, but ranging from a few days to several months, occurred in most but not all cases. This phase was characterized by lability of mood, with various degrees of depression, anxiety, perplexity, and euphoria. Sleep deteriorated markedly, and delusions and hallucinations often appeared. Stauder (1934) stated that such prodromal signs "cannot be distinguished from the beginnings of other schizophrenias" (p. 623).

TABLE 5.1. Clinical Features of Lethal Catatonia

Prodromal phase
   Average duration: 2 weeks
Hyperactive phase
   Average duration: 8 days (1 day to several weeks)
- Extreme motoric excitement
- Refusal of all foods and fluids
- Clouding of consciousness
- Somatic disturbances
- Hyperthermia
Final stage
   Duration less than 4 days
   Stuporous exhaustion (musculature flaccid or rigid, coma, cardiovascular collapse, and death)

An ensuing hyperactive phase began with the development of sustained, intense, and frequently violent motor excitement. Shulack's (1946) account is representative. He described excitement, which increased to:

> a continual maniacal furor, in which the individual will tear off his clothes, tear the clothes to strips, take the bed apart, rip the mattress to pieces, bang and pound almost rhythmically on the walls and windows, dash wildly from the room, assault anyone in reach and run aimlessly and without objective. . . . If placed in restraints, he will strain ceaselessly. (p. 466)

At times, excitement might be interrupted by periods of catatonic stupor and rigidity. Other catatonic signs such as mutism, posturing, echolalia, echopraxia, catalepsy, and staring were often noted during the excited phase. Thought processes became increasingly disorganized and speech became increasingly incoherent. Auditory and visual hallucinations accompanied by bizarre delusions were often prominent. Clouding of consciousness, noted in most cases, was viewed by many authors as one of the cardinal features of the disorder.

Refusal of all foods and fluids was characteristic of the hyperactive phase, leading to cachexia and dehydration. The pulse became rapid, even in periods of momentary rest. Blood pressure was labile, the skin was pale, and perspiration was profuse. Acrocyanosis and spontaneous hematomas of the skin were frequently noted. Hyperthermia, the most striking somatic manifestation, rose rapidly, often attaining levels above 110 °F prior to cessation of excitement. The hyperactive stage of the disorder varied in duration from less than a day to several weeks, but lasted an average of 8 days (Arnold and Stepan 1952).

In the final phase of the disorder, extreme psychomotor excitement gave way to stuporous exhaustion, with extreme hyperthermia followed by cardiovascular collapse, coma, and death. Skeletal muscle tone was often described as "limp" during this terminal stupor (Arnold and Stepan 1952). In other cases, however, muscular rigidity was seen, resembling NMS. Stauder (1934), for instance, observed that after the peak of psychomotor excitement, all 27 patients in his series passed through a stage during which they became extremely rigid and would "lay [sic] in bed with clenched teeth, each muscle tensed" (p. 627) and would exhibit bizarre posturing. In Stauder's (1934) series, terminal rigidity and stupor lasted 36 hours to 4 days. Other authors also described cases presenting initially with motoric excitement and hyperthermia, progressing to protracted stuporous rigidity and death. It must be emphasized that this earlier literature also documented episodes of LC in which the entire clinical course was one of catatonic stupor and rigidity with hyperthermia, unassociated with hyperactivity (Bell 1849; Scheid 1938; Shulack 1944; Tolsma 1956).

Laboratory abnormalities included increased erythrocyte sedimentation rate, blood urea nitrogen, serum potassium and chloride, and decreased calcium. Leukocytosis and lymphopenia were sometimes present. A variety of coagulation abnormalities were variably described.

The syndrome appeared to occur with equal frequency throughout the seasons. Of particular interest was a report by Derby (1933) discussing 187 "manic-depressive exhaustion deaths"; manic patients, compared to patients with stupor, would seem particularly vulnerable to summer heat. This report also indicated a uniform seasonal distribution.

Most early French authors viewed LC as a specific disease rather than a syndrome. They considered LC a special form of encephalitis involving inflammatory and degenerative changes in the central nervous system (CNS). Manifestations of inflammation included lymphocytic and plasmocytic collections around blood vessels. Degenerative lesions were described in the cerebral cortex and subcortical nuclei (Claude and Cuel 1927; Ladame 1919; Redalié 1920). Postmortem findings included satellitosis, ameboid degeneration, and infiltration of large numbers of cells with lipoid material.

In contrast, Kraepelin (1905) and Scheideggar (1929) were among a number of German authors of this period who considered LC a clinical syndrome, comprised of characteristic symptoms and a set course, but lacking a specific etiology. They believed that LC could occur as an outgrowth of various organic diseases as well as in association with functional psychoses. Huber (1954) stated that aside from occurring within the framework of schizophrenia, LC could also develop as a complication of general paresis, brain tumors, cerebrovascular accidents, brain trauma (especially trauma involving the frontal lobe), seizure disorders, various intoxications, and infections. In addition, Huber (1954) mentioned cases of LC "superimposed on unclassifiable brain processes" that presented as an "atypical encephalitis" involving lymphocytic and plasmocytic perivascular infiltrates not unlike those findings described by previous French authors (Claude and Cuel 1927; Ladame 1919; Redalié 1920).

Subsequent to Stauder's (1934) publication, however, LC was increasingly viewed as a functional psychosis, yet Stauder himself never fully dismissed the possibility of an organic etiology. The majority of German authors came to view LC as an outgrowth of schizophrenia. Jahn and Greving (1936), Scheid (1938), and Knoll (1954) felt that they were able to identify schizophrenia in most of their patients who developed LC. Arnold and Stepan (1952) followed 16 survivors of LC for 3 years and found evidence of schizophrenia in 10. However, the remaining six patients were symptom free at follow-up.

The opinion of American authors of this period was more divergent. Malamud and Boyd (1939), Billig and Freeman (1944), and Aronson and Thompson (1950) echoed the German literature, which suggested a decisive link between LC and schizophrenia. In keeping with the line of thought developed by Bell (1849), however, others felt that LC was often an outgrowth of mania. Kraines (1934) focused on the differentiation of acute manic states from organic febrile delirium, but failed to even consider a relationship to schizophrenia. Derby (1933) and Larson (1939) published reports on exhaustion deaths in manic-depressive psychosis and noted that a similar picture could occur in association with schizophrenia. Shulack (1944, 1946) and Davidson (1934) felt that LC could occur with manic-depressive illness, schizophrenia, and postpartum and involutional psychoses as well.

Lack of autopsy findings that could account for the cause of death in LC was emphasized by most German and American authors of the preneuroleptic era. Any CNS abnormalities considered pathonomonic by the French were either unconfirmed or deemed trivial. Postmortem findings were limited to general visceral and encephalic vascular congestion, with some authors noting fibrosis in organs outside the CNS (Bamford and Bean 1932). Histopathologic exam generally revealed nothing more than mild nonspecific degenerative changes, petechiae, and small hemorrhages in the cerebral cortex and other body organs. Bronchopneumonia or other infections found on autopsy were considered "opportunistic" because they occurred in an already exhausted and compromised host. Such infections were "capable of accelerating death but not representing the sole cause of lethal outcome" (Stauder 1934, p. 628). Kraines (1934) summarized controversial autopsy findings by quoting Bell (1849): "slight cerebral and meningal engorgements which constituted the only marks of the disease were no greater than the incidents of sleeplessness, agitation, and death might be expected to leave independent of any great morbid action behind these" (Kraines 1934, p. 38).

Pathophysiologic mechanisms other than inflammatory-degenerative reactions proposed by French authors and noted in some of Huber's (1954) cases were postulated by other authors of this era. Lingjaerde (1963) observed a similarity between the clinical features of LC and those of acute adrenocortical insufficiency: apathy, fatigue, anorexia, and depression followed by the development of psychotic features, clouding of consciousness, hyperthermia, and signs of peripheral vascular collapse often ending in shock and death. In LC, adrenocortical exhaustion was attributed to "excessive physical and mental stress" resulting in "homeostatic chaos" (Lingjaerde 1963, pp. 75–76).

Golse and Morel (1953) compared LC (*delire aigu*) to the "general adaptation syndrome" described by Selye (1956). Selye regarded adrenocortical stimulation as a nonspecific final common pathway of response to diverse physical and mental stressors. He observed that acute outpouring of adrenocortical secretions in response to stress resulted in physical changes such as gastric ulcers. Furthermore, prolonged stress, during which the adrenals functioned with emergency action over extended periods of time, led to a disorder characterized by adrenocortical exhaustion with associated peripheral vascular collapse, shock, and death.

Golse and Morel (1953) noted that, in addition to adrenal exhaustion and peripheral vascular collapse, this end-stage disorder described by Selye shared with LC lesions in the cerebral cortex and hypothalamus such as those mentioned by early French authors. They also observed that *syndrome malin*, like LC and Selye's disorder, involved adrenocortical exhaustion, shock, and characteristic CNS lesions. Also, each could present with "lead-pipe" muscular rigidity. However, *syndrome malin* appeared to differ in its particular association with infections conditions, and, on autopsy, by evidence of extensive inflammatory and degenerative changes within the sympathetic ganglia, to be consistent with diffuse dysfunction of the sympathetic nervous system prior to death.

Other authors posited mechanisms involving more subtle homeostatic abnormalities believed present in psychotic patients, as predisposing to LC, focusing more on autonomic pathways than on endocrine functioning. Adland (1947) referred to studies by Gottlieb and Linder (1935) and others indicating that schizophrenic patients were defective in their homeostatic thermoregulatory capacity. Stauder (1934) cited research suggesting that schizophrenics, particularly of the catatonic subtype, exhibited vasomotor instability. Stauder (1934) thought that this defect correlated with symptoms such as acrocyanosis, labile blood pressure, hematoma of the skin, and increased menstrual blood flow in female patients with LC. Billig and Freeman (1944) discussed preexisting sympathetic nervous system abnormalities in schizophrenics, while Shulack (1946) noted autonomic dysfunction in patients with diverse psychotic conditions going on to develop LC.

Finally, Adland (1947) viewed LC as a "psychogenic illness originating in a need for selfannihilation as a solution to a problem" (p. 66). He reviewed literature indicating that high fever, leukocytosis, and vascular collapse may occur as isolated symptoms on a purely functional basis. Adland speculated that in LC these symptoms erupted in unison. He believed that in patients who developed LC "the autonomic nervous system may be the most vulnerable of the organ systems" (Adlund 1947, p. 64). In addition to somatic treatments, Adland advocated a strong positive doctor/patient relationship, even when the patient appears confused and distant.

Contemporary Literature

To assess the current status of LC, we identified a series of 292 cases of LC reported since 1960 (Mann et al. 1986). A number of the contemporary reports from which the series of 292 cases were drawn will now be discussed, with emphasis on publications involving a substantial number of cases. Most reports view LC as a syndrome associated with both functional and organic conditions, as shown in Table 5.2. Reports viewing LC as confined to the functional psychoses will be considered first.

Sedivec (1981) reported eight patients with LC treated between 1970 and 1979. Each case involved acute psychosis with psychomotor agitation, confusion, and hyperthermia, progressing to exhaustion and stupor. In one case, stupor advanced to coma and death. Each was considered the outgrowth of a mood disorder diagnosed as mania in four cases, and agitated melancholia in the other four. Seven of eight patients survived, attributed to timely intervention with electroconvulsive therapy (ECT). On autopsy, the one fatality showed no primary brain pathology. Cerebrospinal fluid (CSF) and viral studies were negative.

TABLE 5.2. Disorders Associated with Lethal Catatonia Syndrome

Functional psychiatric disorders
  Schizophrenia
  Mood disorders
  Periodic catatonia
  "Atypical psychosis"
Cerebrovascular disorders
  Basilar artery thrombosis
  Bilateral hemorrhagic infarction of anterior cingulate gyri
  Bilateral hemorrhagic lesions of temporal lobes
Tumors
  Periventricular diffuse pinealoma
  Glioma of the third ventricle
  Glioma involving the splenum of the corpus callosum
  Angioma of the midbrain
Head trauma
  Closed head trauma
  Surgical removal of lesions near the hypothalamus
Infections
  Viral encephalitis
  Typhoid fever
  Malaria
  General paresis
  Viral hepatitis
  Bacterial septicemia
Seizure disorders
  Autonomic (diencephalic) epilepsy
  Petit mal status
Metabolic disorders
  Hyperthyroidism
  Addison's disease
  Cushing's disease
  Uremia
  Wernicke's encephalopathy
  Cerebral anoxia
Toxic disorders
  Postoperative states
  Tetraethyl lead poisoning
  Sedative-hypnotic withdrawal
  Neuroleptic malignant syndrome

Note. Adapted from Mann et al. (1986), with permission.

Häfner and Kasper (1982) reported 10 cases of LC treated between 1975 and 1981. Two patients presented with catatonic excitement, four were stuporous, and four had features of both stupor and excitement. The first two patients in their series—one excited and the other stuporous—received only neuroleptics and supportive measures. Both died and in neither could autopsy findings account for the cause of death. The next seven patients were treated with ECT and attained remission following two to 14 treatments. In the case of the tenth patient who presented with catatonia and fever (38.6 °C), temperature elevation was attributed to bronchopneumonia rather than LC. All patients in this series were considered schizophrenic.

Laskowska and associates studied 55 patients hospitalized in Poland between 1951 and 1960, each of whom displayed a febrile catatonic picture consistent with "Stauder's lethal catatonia." Many of the findings from this study were published in English (Laskowska et al. 1965). Forty-nine cases involved catatonic excitement with features of delirium. The remaining six cases were characterized by stupor and hyperthermia. Patients treated in the later part of the decade received neuroleptics. Thirty-five patients survived, and 32 of these were followed for 2 to 12 years. On follow-up, 27 (84 percent) of 32 patients exhibited signs of chronic schizophrenia. In the remaining five patients, no abnormalities were noted after 3 to 5 years, although the authors suggested that further observation would be necessary before concluding that these individuals were truly free of schizophrenia. In this series, 20 of the 55 patients eventually died; 10 came to autopsy. The gross autopsy findings were considered minimal and insufficient to account for the fulminating, fatal course. Cardiac enlargement, found in all patients, and bronchopneumonia, present in four patients, were felt to represent nonspecific complications. While at least one-third of patients received an initial diagnosis suggesting an organic condition, the authors believed that neither encephalitis nor any other organic condition could be causative in those cases that received a full evaluation on follow-up or at autopsy. They concluded that "Stauder's type of catatonia" was an outgrowth of schizophrenia. However, they mentioned that it was difficult to account for temperature elevations and for certain laboratory abnormalities, including albuminuria (22 cases), elevated blood urea nitrogen (nine cases), increased urinary urobilinogen (24 cases), and elevated erythrocyte sedimentation rate (many cases). In particular, they noted the obscure origin of CSF changes in a small number of cases: increased CSF protein in one case, 51 lymphocytes in one fatal case, and up to 34 lymphocytes in two nonfatal cases. They observed that similar CSF abnormalities had been reported previously in LC and had puzzled other investigators.

Gabris and Muller (1983) reported 14 cases of "catatonie pernicieuse": four presented as agitated, eight were stuporous, and two exhibited a mixture of agitation and stupor. Elevations in hepatic transaminases, erythrocyte sedimentation rate, and serum glucose were noted. Thirteen patients were treated with neuroleptics; six received ECT in addition to neuroleptic treatment. In 13 patients, LC was viewed as an outgrowth of schizophrenia. In the 14th patient LC was viewed as a consequence of cerebral anoxia rather than schizophrenia. This patient was treated only with respiratory analeptics and responded favorably. The two patients in this series who died received only neuroleptics (not ECT). In both, death was attributed to cardiac insufficiency. Interestingly, one patient's improvement coincided with the discontinuation of neuroleptics; an "excess of neuroleptics" was considered as a possible cause of death in another patient. Gabris and Muller's (1983) observation that LC could occur as an outgrowth of cerebral anoxia is consistent with the views of a number of contemporary investigators who, like Kraepelin (1905) and Scheideggar (1929), believed that LC is a syndrome associated with both functional and organic etiologies.

Molokov (1962), who reported 38 patients with LC treated in the Soviet Union, identified 11 cases in which a preexisting organic condition appeared to have initiated the full syndromal picture of LC. Seven cases were believed to be due to bacterial septicemia that evolved from endometritis (four cases) and aortitis (one case). In the remaining two cases, the source of infection could not be identified. Additional causes of LC included one case of general paresis, two cases of cerebrovascular thrombosis, and one case following tetraethyl lead poisoning.

Schmidt and Zacher (1974) conducted a retrospective chart review of 50 LC cases treated between 1950 and 1970; all but seven ended in death. Clinically, these patients closely resembled those described in the earlier literature: 56 percent presented initially with excitement and 14 percent exhibited excitement alternating with stupor. Only 10 percent were uniformly stuporous throughout their clinical course. The remainder were characterized as "catatonias with posturing and stereotypes" (Schmidt and Zacher 1974, p. 68). The majority of patients in this series received neuroleptics; half received ECT. After excluding 10 patients who were not autopsied (three who died and seven who survived), Schmidt and Zacher divided the remaining 40 into three groups. Group 1 contained 23 patients, each of whom failed to exhibit significant pathologic findings on autopsy. Patients in this group were considered to represent "genuine" functional LC. Group 2 consisted of six patients in whom a preexisting organic illness was believed to have initiated the full LC syndrome. Preexisting illnesses included viral encephalitis (two cases), bacterial septicemia evolving from endocarditis, myocarditis, and cholangitis (single cases), and a final case attributed to uremia. The 11 patients in Group 3 had autopsy findings that were secondarily associated with catatonic inmobility such as deep venous thrombosis and pulmonary embolus and were implicated in causing death. Schmidt and Zacher differentiated these Group 3 cases from "genuine" LC and considered them benign catatonia rendered fatal by severe intercurrent medical complications. They emphasized, however, that prior to postmortem exam, the three groups had not been distinguished on clinical grounds, and all cases had originally been considered "genuine" functional LC.

Penn et al. (1972) described a 25-year-old man with no previous psychiatric history who, following a prodromal period involving 2 weeks of mounting psychopathology, was hospitalized in a violent, excited, and confused state. Despite administration of neuroleptics and a course of six ECT treatments started on hospital day 4, he continued to exhibit excitement and assaultiveness, alternating with periods of posturing and waxy flexibility, during which he maintained a fixed position for hours. Although there were no localizing signs on neurologic exam, and all studies (including blood cultures and radiologic findings) were normal, results of lumbar punctures on days 6 and 7 revealed 18 white blood cells (17 lymphocytes) and nine white blood cells (all lymphocytes), respectively. An electroencephalogram (EEG) could not be done on this patient. Temperature elevations developed on day 3 and ultimately reached 41.7 °C. Exhaustion intervened and the patient became hypotensive and died on the ninth hospital day. This apparent classic picture of excited lethal catatonia was attributed to viral encephalitis.

Morant (1984) reported a similar case of violent catatonic excitement followed by stupor, hyperthermia, and death. Although three lumbar punctures over a 2-week period showed normal CSF pressure, protein, and glucose, and although serum and CSF studies for viruses, fungi, and bacteria were negative, the CSF contained progressive numbers of lymphocytes—24, 29, and $41/mm^3$—suggesting a viral encephalitis. On autopsy, however, numerous sections of the brain exhibited "minimal pathology," except for an area of neurophagia in the pons.

As noted previously, two cases in Schmidt and Zacher's (1974) series were believed to be due to viral encephalitis. In addition, Miyoshi et al. (1968) and Ishii et al. (1972) reported cases of LC that were attributed to lymphocytic meningo-encephalitis on autopsy. Koziel-Schminda (1973) reported additional similar cases. It is known that various types of viral encephalitis may present with psychiatric symptoms prior to the onset of focal neurologic findings, EEG changes, and CSF abnormalities (Wilson 1976). Furthermore, on autopsy, microscopic changes may be so subtle as to go unrecognized.

Retrospective Review

In our review (Mann et al. 1986) of 292 cases of LC, 265 came from 20 reports representative of more than 50 recent publications by foreign authors. The remaining 27 cases were reported in 12 articles found in an exhaustive search of the post-1960 North American literature. Fifteen of these 27 American cases came from a single study that provided little specific data (Bohorfoush et al. 1965). It should be emphasized that most patients received neuroleptics at some point during their treatment. We compared epidemiologic and descriptive parameters of recent cases of LC to cases from the preneuroleptic era.

In 279 cases where sex was specified, 187 (67 percent) were female. In the earlier literature there was a 4:1 female to male ratio. This indicates that women continue to be more commonly affected, although this trend may now be slightly reduced. Of the 292, 176 (60 percent) died, indicating that this disorder remains quite deadly, although relatively less lethal than in the earlier era when mortality ranged from 75 to 100 percent. The mean age of occurrence was 33 years in the more recent group compared to 25 years in the preneuroleptic era. Division into age cohorts showed 16 percent were younger than age 20, 30 percent were age 20 to 29, 20 percent were age 30 to 39, 21 percent were age 40 to 49, 10 percent were age 50 to 60, and 3 percent were over age 60. The wide age distribution contrasted with the belief of some early authors that LC occurs primarily in the second and third decades of life. Similar to findings from the preneuroleptic era, a uniform seasonal distribution was evident.

Overall, 36 (12 percent) from the sample of 292 contemporary LC cases were believed to be organic in origin, as in Schmidt and Zacher's (1974) Group 2. The most common disorders were viral encephalitis and septicemia. These are to be differentiated from cases described in Schmidt and Zacher's (1974) Group 3, which consisted of benign catatonias rendered deadly by pulmonary embolism and other consequences of catatonic immobility, such as refusal of fluids and nutrients. It should be noted that a number of reports from which the 292 cases were drawn had excluded cases of LC with a suspected or confirmed organic etiology. Thus the 12 percent figure found in our sample may underestimate the frequency with which lethal catatonias of this type occur.

Of the 292 cases, 256 (88 percent) were considered the outgrowth of various functional psychotic disorders as indicated in Table 5.2. Of these 256 cases of functional LC, 154 (60 percent) cases ended in death. Autopsy data were available for 92. Of these 92 cases, 72 (78 percent) proved autopsy negative, and as such would fall into Schmidt and Zacher's (1974) Group 1 as "genuine" functional LC. The remaining 20, however, exhibited specific postmortem findings related to catatonic immobility, which could account for death and would fall into Schmidt and Zacher's Group 3.

The "classic" hyperactive form involving extreme motoric excitement and progressive hyperthermia prior to the onset of stupor continued to predominate with 69 percent of cases presenting in this fashion. However, 31 percent of patients exhibited a primarily stuporous course. This represents a change from the earlier era, when only about 10 percent of cases involved a primarily stuporous course. In many of these cases involving a primarily stuporous course, stupor and hyperthermia developed only following the initiation of neuroleptic treatment, giving rise to questions concerning the demarcation of LC from NMS.

On casual inspection, those LC cases occurring during neuroleptic treatment in which stupor is preceded by a classic stage of extreme motoric excitement seem to resemble NMS, since NMS may be preceded by hyperactivity (Itoh et al. 1977; Schibuk and Schacter 1986). However, the excitement seen in NMS prior to the onset of stupor is unassociated with the dramatically progressive temperature elevations characteristic of the excited stage of classic LC (Mann and Caroff 1987). Rather, in NMS, hyperthermia usually emerges with the onset of stupor and akinesia. Thus classic LC that presents with initial excitement may be distinguishable from NMS on clinical grounds on the basis of a well-documented history of extreme hyperthermia present in the excited phase.

However, we were able to identify 65 patients (22 percent) from the 292 recent LC cases whose clinical phenomenology appeared equally consistent with a diagnosis of NMS. These were patients who developed a hyperthermic catatonic stupor during neuroleptic treatment, and who, if initially excited, had been free of significant hyperthermia during that excitement. Thus 22 percent of the contemporary LC cases do, in fact, appear indistinguishable from NMS. Viewing LC as a syndrome that may occur as an outgrowth of both organic and functional disorders, we have suggested that NMS represents a neuroleptic-induced iatrogenic form of organic LC (Mann et al. 1986). Accordingly, the emergence of NMS as a subtype of LC could help explain the increased percentage of LC cases involving a primarily stuporous course reported in the contemporary world literature.

Finally, our review suggests that the prevalence of LC has probably declined worldwide since the advent of modern psychopharmacologic agents. This decline may be largely attributable to the efficacy of such agents in treating underlying disorders before they progress into LC. However, lack of familiarity with LC probably accounts for the particular scarcity of recent American reports.

Pathogenesis

The pathogenesis of LC, both functional and organic types, remains poorly understood. The diverse causes of LC (see Table 5.2) suggest the involvement of multiple neuroanatomic loci and possibly multiple neurotransmitter systems. However, in view of hyperthermia and marked autonomic changes, most workers have considered the hypothalamus as a major locus of involvement.

Kick (1981) viewed LC as catatonia complicated by "central diencephalic dysregulatory hyperthermia" (p. 19). This type of hyperthermia involved pale skin, profuse perspiration, increased muscle tone, and, with ongoing deterioration of diencephalic functioning, severe tachycardia, lability of blood pressure, and cyanosis. Kick (1981) believed that central diencephalic dysregulatory hyperthermia also developed in association with NMS.

Similarly, Stoudemire and Luther (1984) and Fricchione (1985) suggested that LC may represent psychogenic catatonia complicated by a "hypothalamic crisis," accounting for hyperthermia and autonomic changes. In addition, both authors speculated that a parallel relationship may exist between neuroleptic-induced catatonia (without hyperthermia) and NMS, namely, that NMS may represent neuroleptic-induced catatonia also complicated by a hypothalamic crisis. Fricchione (1985) stated: "Perhaps NMS is to neuroleptic-induced catatonia as lethal catatonia is to psychogenic catatonia . . . neuroleptic-induced catatonia may end in NMS, just as psychogenic catatonia may result in lethal catatonia" (p. 306).

Tolsma (1967) also focused on dysfunction of hypothalamic homeostatic mechanisms in the etiology of LC. He suggested that many of the behavioral and somatic abnormalities characteristic of LC could be attributed to an abnormal reaction of the hypothalamic-pituitary-adrenal axis in response to various organic and psychogenic stressors. In addition, Tolsma (1967) noted that disturbances of the hypothalamus, by virtue of its connections with other CNS structures such as the hippocampus, amygdaloid nucleus, and, in particular, the reticular-activating system (RAS) may account for the diverse neuropsychiatric symptoms seen in LC.

The possibility that dysfunction of the mesencephalic-diencephalic RAS or its rostral projections may contribute to the pathogenesis of LC is of considerable interest. Akinetic mutism, a disorder that should not be confused with "coma vigil" (Ross and Stewart 1981), involves severe hypomotility, diminished arousal, and mutism, and has at times presented clinically indistinguishable from psychogenic catatonia (Barris and Schuman 1953; Cairns 1952; Cravioto et al. 1960; Sours 1962). Akinetic mutism has generally been attributed to partial damage of the mesencephalic-diencephalic RAS, or of RAS projections to the anterior cingulate gyrus, a cortical area particularly suited to influence the hypothalamus and to integrate the "emotional components" of cognition (Papez 1937; Weinberger 1987). Furthermore, certain cases of akinetic mutism have been associated with the full LC syndrome. Such cases have followed bilateral lesions of the anterior cingulate gyrus (Barris and Schuman 1953), various hypothalamic lesions including damage to the mammillary bodies and periventricular hypothalamic nuclei (Schilder 1934), damage to other areas near the third ventricle (Cairns 1952; Newmann 1955), and various brain-stem lesions (Cravioto et al. 1960).

Recently, a direct route from the brain-stem RAS to the anterior cingulate gyri involving a midbrain dopaminergic projection has been clarified in the rat (Lindvall and Björklund 1982) (see Figure 5.1). This projection passes rostrally in the medial forebrain bundle, coursing in proximity to the lateral hypothalamus and globus pallidus, ending in the anterior cingulate gyrus. The anatomic location of this route and the anatomic distribution of lesions associated with akinetic mutism appear consistent with a pathogenic role for interruption of this dopaminergic pathway in causing mutism, diminished arousal, hypokinesia, and, in some cases, abnormalities in limbic/hypothalamic regulatory mechanisms in akinetic mutism, and by extension, LC. Wambebe and Osuide (1982) have summarized further data supporting a role for endogenous dopamine in mediating arousal. As in NMS,

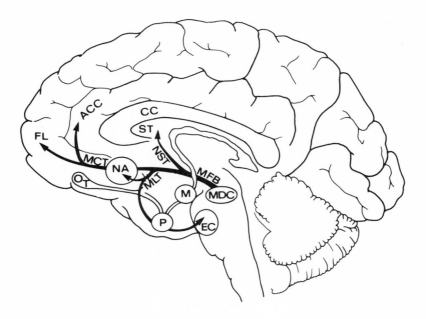

ACC – Anterior Cingulate Cortex	MFB – Medial Forebrain Bundle
CC – Corpus Callosum	MLT – Mesolimbic Tract
EC – Entorhinal Cortex	NA – Nucleus Accumbens Septi
FL – Frontal Lobe	NST – Nigrostrial Tract
M – Mammillary Body	OB(OT) – Olfactory Tract and Bulb
MCT – Mesocortical Tract	P – Pituitary
MDC – Midbrain Dopaminergic Cells	ST – Striatum

Figure 5.1. Direct route from brainstem reticular-activating system to anterior cingulate gyrus involving dopamine projections ascending in medial forebrain bundle.

187

some patients with akinetic mutism may be responsive to the administration of direct dopamine agonists such as bromocriptine (Ross and Stewart 1981). Several other lines of evidence suggest that altered dopaminergic transmission in other brain areas could account for many of the symptoms seen in LC. The proposed alterations in dopamine systems parallel those believed to occur in NMS, where neuroleptic-induced dopamine receptor blockade appears to have a causal role (see Chapter 1).

When catecholaminergic neurons were first identified, major cell groups were designated as A1 through A16, based on their caudorostral ascending order, with groups in the mid and rostral brain areas (A8 through A16) being exclusively dopaminergic (Moore 1987) (Figure 5.2). Although midbrain

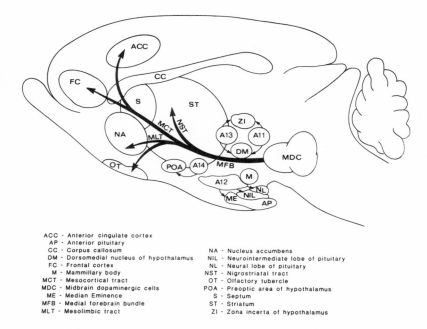

ACC - Anterior cingulate cortex
AP - Anterior pituitary
CC - Corpus callosum
DM - Dorsomedial nucleus of hypothalamus
FC - Frontal cortex
M - Mammillary body
MCT - Mesocortical tract
MDC - Midbrain dopaminergic cells
ME - Median Eminence
MFB - Medial forebrain bundle
MLT - Mesolimbic tract

NA - Nucleus accumbens
NIL - Neurointermediate lobe of pituitary
NL - Neural lobe of pituitary
NST - Nigrostriatal tract
OT - Olfactory tubercle
POA - Preoptic area of hypothalamus
S - Septum
ST - Striatum
ZI - Zona incerta of hypothalamus

Figure 5.2. Hypothalamic dopamine neurons and their projections in the rat. Ascending midbrain dopamine pathways are also indicated.

dopaminergic neurons giving rise to ascending mesencephalic dopaminergic projections are no longer considered separated into discrete A8, A9, and A10 dopamine cell groups, but are viewed as forming an overlapping continuum supplying dopamine innervation throughout the forebrain (Robbins and Everitt 1982; Roth et al. 1987), their distribution patterns are generally described using the original terms: mesocortical, mesolimbic, and nigrostriatal dopaminergic projections.

In addition to the mesocortical dopaminergic pathway to the anterior cingulate gyrus discussed above, a mesocortical pathway to the prefrontal cortex has also been described (Figures 5.1 and 5.2). While severe stress is associated with generalized activation of dopaminergic systems in animals, the prefrontal mesocortical dopaminergic system appears to be unique in responding to stress that is mild or experiential, for example, conditioned fear (Roth et al. 1987; Weinberger 1987). Furthermore, the prefrontal cortex exerts feedback control of mesolimbic dopamine activity, probably through inhibition of mesencephalic dopamine neurons, and increased prefrontal mesocortical dopamine activity during stress could result in decreased mesolimbic and nigrostriatal dopamine transmission.

The mesolimbic dopaminergic pathway, believed to be involved in psychosis, courses through the medial forebrain bundle to innervate mesolimbic areas such as the nucleus accumbens, olfactory tubercles, septum, and amygdala. Reduced mesolimbic dopaminergic transmission to the nucleus accumbens appears to result in akinesia and catalepsy (Anden and Johnels 1977). Rigidity, however, which occurs when both agonists and antagonists muscle groups receive continuous positive feedback, may involve the nigrostriatal dopaminergic pathway (Anden and Johnels 1977; Pearlman 1986). Movement-related inhibitory output from the neostriatum to the medial globus pallidus and the substantia nigra pars reticulata is conveyed by striatal neurons that utilize gamma-aminobutyric acid (GABA) as their neurotransmitter (Penney and Young 1983). The substantia nigra pars reticulata and medial globus pallidus act together as a single nucleus and represent a major outflow tract from the basal ganglia to the thalamocortical cells involved in regulating muscle tone (Schultz 1987). Reduced mesostriatal dopaminergic transmission could inhibit GABAergic transmission from striatum to medial globus pallidus and substantia nigra pars reticulata, thus disinhibiting the ventral anterior and ventral lateral nuclei of the thalamus and their projections to prefrontal cortex and ultimately motor cortex with resultant rigidity (Penney and Young 1983; Starr et al. 1983).

Dopaminergic neurons located in the hypothalamus have been divided into two major groups: the incertohypothalamic dopaminergic system with cell bodies in areas A11, A13, and A14; and the tuberohypophysial system with dopaminergic neurons in the A12 area (Moore 1987) (see Figure 5.2). Incertohypothalamic dopaminergic neurons located in the periventricular region of the anterior hypothalamus (A14) appear to innervate the medial preoptic hypothalamus, the key locus involved in dopaminergic-mediated heat loss (see Chapter 2). In the rat, tuberohypophysial dopaminergic neurons (A12) are located primarily in the arcuate nucleus and project to the neural and neurointermediate lobes of the pituitary, as well as to the median eminence.

The tuberohypophysial dopaminergic system also exerts a tonic inhibitory influence on pituitary release of beta-endorphin, an endogenous opiate with thermoregulatory effects (Clark 1979), and whose injection into the rat CSF is associated with catatonic rigidity, immobility, and maintenance of awkward postures as well as hypotension, bradycardia, and respiratory depression (Sandyk 1985b). During stress, beta-endorphin secretion from the pituitary is accompanied by secretion of adrenocorticotropic hormone (ACTH), consistent with both having a common precursor molecule contained in pituitary secretory granules (Guillemin 1985). In severely stressful states such as bacterial septicemia (an organic cause of lethal catatonia), release of beta-endorphin may account for autonomic changes that eventuate in shock, while onset of shock could be buffered by concurrent release of endogenous ACTH. Also, similar mechanisms might be involved in the reported efficacy of exogenous ACTH and corticosteroids in treating LC as reviewed in this chapter. As noted in Chapter 2, in addition to intrinsic hypothalamic neurons, projections from mesencephalic dopaminergic systems to the hypothalamus have been identified (Javoy-Agid et al. 1984), although their role in hypothalamic regulation and regulation of other autonomic functions remains unclear (Gonzalez et al. 1986).

Disturbances in a recently identified diencephalospinal dopaminergic pathway might also contribute to autonomic disregulation (Lindvall et al. 1983) (see Chapter 1). This pathway originates from dopamine neurons located periventricularly in the dorsal hypothalamus, posterior hypothalamus, and caudal thalamus (A11), and provides dopaminergic innvervation to the intermediolateral spinal column mediating inhibition of preganglionic sympathetic neurons. Thus abnormalities in this pathway could account for signs of increased sympathetic activation characteristic of LC.

Peripheral dopamine receptors (Goldberg et al. 1986) may also mediate dopaminergic influences on autonomic regulatory mechanisms. Two subtypes of peripheral dopamine receptors have been identified: peripheral dopamine-1, for postsynaptic receptors subserving relaxation of smooth muscle, and peripheral dopamine-2 receptors located on postganglionic sympathetic neurons that inhibit norepinephrine release from sympathetic nerve terminals, leading to peripheral vasodilation and decreased heart rate. Also, recent evidence has indicated the existence of peripheral dopamine circulating in plasma, primarily in conjugated form and principally derived from peripheral sympathetic nerve terminals (Yoneda et al. 1985). Similar to the diencephalospinal dopaminergic pathway, dysfunction in peripheral dopamine mechanisms could cause autonomic instability and promote the development of a "hyperadrenergic state." Additional support for the involvement of dopamine in the pathogenesis of LC is provided by theories implicating dopaminergic dysfunction in schizophrenia and mania, the two functional psychotic conditions most commonly associated with LC.

This discussion has focused primarily on the possible involvement of dopaminergic systems in the pathogenesis of lethal catatonia. However, as in NMS, dopaminergic transmission would probably be influenced and regulated by diverse neurotransmitter systems such as those mentioned above, (GABA, endogenous opiods, and catecholamines involved in "hyperadrenergia") as well as others implicated in the pathogenesis of NMS and similar drug-induced conditions discussed in Chapters 1 and 3. Furthermore, similar to NMS, factors involved in the pathogenesis of LC probably include changes in neuromuscular function and, at the postsynaptic molecular level, alterations in second messenger functioning.

Along these lines a role for disordered calcium regulation in the pathogenesis of LC has also been suggested. Carman and Wyatt (1977) described a 47-year-old man with periodic episodes of psychotic agitation lasting 4 days, alternating with 4-day periods of catatonic stupor. During every third complete cycle (i.e., every 24 days), his agitation progressed to "a frenetic delirium with tremulous muscular rigidity, piloerection, mutism, bizarre posturing, and hyperthermia with oral temperatures above 40 °C" (Carman and Wyatt 1977, p. 1124). Hyperthermic episodes were associated with elevations in serum calcium and creatine phosphokinase (CPK). Furthermore, injection of synthetic salmon calcitonin, which diminishes serum calcium levels, aborted these episodes.

Patients exhibiting periodic exacerbations of psychotic agitation often have increased serum calcium accompanied by a reciprocal decrease in CSF calcium (Carman and Wyatt 1979; Carman et al. 1984). Decreased calcium in hypothalamic thermoregulatory centers has been shown to cause hyperthermia in the above case. Furthermore, increased myoplasmic calcium consequent to increased serum calcium could result in muscular rigidity and CPK elevation. By lowering serum calcium, calcitonin may promote sequestration of muscle calcium from cytoplasm to mitochondria reducing muscular rigidity and CPK elevation, while calcitonin-induced increase in CSF calcium may reduce hyperthermia (Carman and Wyatt 1977; Carman et al. 1984). Recently, Kaufmann and Wyatt (1987) have emphasized that both calcium and cyclic AMP "represent interdependent intracellular messengers" linked to DA receptors and that understanding of their interactions could "provide both a necessary and sufficient explanation for NMS and related conditions" including LC (Kaufmann and Wyatt, 1987; p. 1426).

Treatment

Functional Lethal Catatonia

While neuroleptics may often prevent the development of LC by treating underlying functional disorders, they appear largely ineffective in halting the syndrome once in its full-blown form. Yet two recent reports provide some support for the use of neuroleptics in treating patients with early signs of LC and hyperthermia less than 38 °C. Laskowska and Chrzanowicz (1967), in an uncontrolled clinical trial, used trifluoperazine, 10 to 30 mg daily, in 13 patients with hyperactive or stuporous catatonia and body temperature ranging from 37.1 to 38.2 °C. All patients responded favorably. Häfner and Kasper (1983) felt that LC detected early, with body temperature below 38 °C, in the absence of severe autonomic disturbances, could be adequately treated with large doses of high-potency neuroleptics, for example, 20 to 90 mg haloperidol daily. However, neuroleptic treatment was abandoned in favor of ECT when hyperthermia exceeded 38 °C.

In contrast, other authors have suggested that neuroleptics may aggravate episodes of LC (Chrisstoffels and Thiel

1970; Gabris and Muller 1983; Maitre et al. 1982); as in NMS, where stopping neuroleptic treatment is mandatory and continuation is associated with increased morbidity and the likelihood of a fatal outcome. Furthermore, neuroleptics may be less effective than ECT in the treatment of functional catatonia (Abrams and Taylor 1976). The delay in onset of action of neuroleptics may allow the disorder to progress to malnutrition, dehydration, and fever, heralding LC.

In view of the questionable efficacy of neuroleptics, and in order to exclude aggravating or confounding effects of these drugs, the first step in the management of catatonic patients who develop hyperthermia should be to discontinue neuroleptics. This should be followed by an extensive medical evaluation and other measures as discussed for NMS in Chapter 1. Most patients with the full LC syndrome will require parenteral fluid support. The severe autonomic symptomatology and the high incidence of medical complications dictate early medical consultation and interdisciplinary treatment, preferably in an intensive care unit.

Although controlled studies are lacking, existing data indicate that ECT may be an effective and practical treatment for LC when it occurs as an outgrowth of a functional psychiatric disturbance. Several clinicians have reported excellent recovery rates with the use of ECT (Häfner and Kasper 1982; Sedivec 1981). However, ECT appears to be effective only if it is initiated before severe progression of symptoms. The development of a comatose state or a temperature in excess of 41 °C augurs poorly for functional LC responding even to ECT. Arnold and Stepan (1952) found that in 19 patients starting ECT within 5 days of the onset of hyperthermia, 16 survived, whereas in 14 patients who began treatment beyond this point, ECT had no effect in preventing death.

While earlier protocols for ECT treatment of LC called for particularly intensive treatment—for example, four treatments in the first 24 hours (Arnold and Stepan 1952)—recent trials with ECT have indicated that it can be successful when given once daily or every other day for a total of five to 15 treatments (usually unilateral), often with substantial improvement after only one to four treatments (Häfner and Kasper 1982; Sedivic 1981).

Several European authors have suggested that ACTH and corticosteroids are equally effective as ECT in treating LC and that these agents are possibly safer given the poor physical condition of most patients with LC (Chrisstoffels and Thiel 1970; Lingjaerde 1963). However, since severely debilitated patients with LC have generally tolerated ECT without incident, and since the utility of hormone therapy is less well documented, ECT appears to be the preferred treatment. ACTH and corticosteroids may be used if ECT proves ineffective.

A few cases of LC have been successfully treated with artificial hibernation, that is, the pharmacologic induction of hypothermia (Fisher and Greiner 1960; Neveu et al. 1973). However, this procedure is hazardous and should probably be avoided. Furthermore, it employs phenothiazines, which may worsen the clinical picture. Finally, Kaufmann and Wyatt (1987) have advocated the use of benzodiazepines in treating LC, and, in addition, have suggested that calcitonin might be effective.

Organic Lethal Catatonia

In LC occurring as an outgrowth of an organic process, treatment must obviously be directed at the underlying condition. Nevertheless, anecdotal reports have described ECT as dramatically effective and at times life-saving as a symptomatic measure in catatonic and delirious states complicated by a wide variety of illnesses (Breakly and Kala 1977; Roberts 1963). Roberts (1963) felt that in these cases the efficacy of ECT was largely independent of the underlying condition but that improvement was likely to be transient if the organic illness persisted. While any conclusions from these cases must be regarded as speculative, observations suggest that ECT has the potential to arrest fulminating LC-like confusional syndromes that complicate various organic conditions, thus preventing death and allowing permanent recovery if the underlying condition remits spontaneously or can be corrected.

ECT may also be helpful in drug-induced forms of LC, such as NMS (see Chapter 1). In NMS, however, dantrolene and dopamine agonists may have more specific therapeutic effects and may be more practical as an initial therapeutic intervention, with ECT held in ready reserve.

Conclusion

LC is a life-threatening hyperthermic neuropsychiatric disorder described long before the introduction of neuroleptic drugs. A review of the world literature on LC has indicated that although the prevalence of the disorder may have declined, it continues to occur, as reported primarily in the foreign literature. Lack of recognition probably accounts for the paucity of reported cases in recent North American literature. Failure to recognize LC has significant clinical implications. Once developed, this disorder assumes an autonomous and frequently fatal course independent of its etiology.

Recent findings and findings from the preneuroleptic era suggest that LC represents a syndrome rather than a specific disease. LC may be caused by diverse organic disorders as well as functional psychiatric disturbances. From this perspective, NMS may be considered a neuroleptic-induced iatrogenic or toxic form of LC. However, those initially excited cases of LC that progress to rigidity and catatonic stupor during the course of neuroleptic treatment may be distinguishable from NMS on the basis of well-documented, extreme hyperthermia during the excited phase. Other cases of LC that follow a primarily stuporous course with rigidity and hyperthermia following the initiation of neuroleptic treatment appear indistinguishable from NMS. This distinction is not always clear, however, and in many cases the question of LC or NMS may be unanswerable.

Although the pathogenesis of LC remains poorly understood, disordered functioning within the diencephalon and other brain areas appears likely, possibly involving alterations of central dopaminergic transmission. ECT appears to be the preferred treatment for LC stemming from functional psychotic conditions and perhaps even in cases related to underlying physical disorders. However, it is imperative in the latter instance to identify and correct the underlying disorder. Neuroleptics appear generally inadequate in treating LC and, in fact, may aggravate or complicate episodes of the disorder.

In this book, we have considered diverse human hyperthermic syndromes resembling NMS that have been recently described as complications of treatment with modern psychopharmacologic agents. These reactions may overlap clinically with each other and may share common pathophysiologic mechanisms. As discussed in Chapter 1, Delay and associates' use of the term *syndrome malin des neuroleptiques* evolved from their perception of NMS as a neuroleptic-induced subtype of a more general syndrome malin. As such, syndrome malin appears to overlap conceptually with LC; both define a human hyperthermic syndrome classically associated with functional and organic illnesses and, more recently, recognized in association with contemporary psychopharmacologic treatment.

References

Abrams R, Taylor MA: Catatonia: a prospective clinical study. Arch Gen Psychiatry 33:579–581, 1976

Abrams R, Taylor MA: EEG observations during combined lithium and neuroleptic treatment. Am J Psychiatry 136:336–337, 1979

Abreo K, Shelp WD, Kosself A, et al: Amoxapine-associated rhabdomyolysis and acute renal failure: case report. J Clin Psychiatry 43:426–427, 1982

Addonizio G: Rapid induction of extrapyramidal side effects with combined use of lithium and neuroleptics. J Clin Psychopharmacol 5:296–298, 1985

Addonizio G, Susman VL: ECT as a treatment alternative for patients with symptoms of neuroleptic malignant syndrome. J Clin Psychiatry 48:102–105, 1987

Addonizio G, Susman VL, Roth SD: Symptoms of neuroleptic malignant syndrome in 82 consecutive inpatients. Am J Psychiatry 143:1587–1590, 1986

Addonizio G, Susman VL, Roth SD: Neuroleptic malignant syndrome: review and analysis of 115 cases. Biol Psychiatry 22:1004–1020, 1987

Addy RO, Foliart RH, Saran AS, et al: EEG observations during combined haloperidol-lithium treatment. Biol Psychiatry 21:170–176, 1986

Adityanjee, Singh S, Singh G, et al: Spectrum concept of neuroleptic malignant syndrome. Br J Psychiatry 153:107–111, 1988.

Adland ML: Review, case studies, therapy and interpretation of the acute exhaustive psychoses. Psychiatr Q 21:38–69, 1947

Ahern CP: Electrical stimulation triggers porcine malignant hyperthermia. Res Vet Sci 39:257–258, 1985

Aizenberg D, Shalev A, Munitz H: The aftercare of the patient with the neuroleptic malignant syndrome. Br J Psychiatry 146:317–318, 1985

Akhtar S, Buckman J: The differential diagnosis of mutism: a review and report of 3 unusual cases. Diseases of the Nervous System 38:558–563, 1977

Alevizos B: Toxic reactions to lithium and neuroleptics. Br J Psychiatry 135:482–483, 1979

Allan RN, White HC: Side effects of parenteral long-acting phenothiazines. Br Med J 1:221, 1972

Allen RM: Role of amantadine in the management of neuroleptic-induced extrapyramidal syndrome: overview and pharmacology. Clin Neuropharmacol 6(Suppl 1):64–73, 1983

Allison JH, Boshaus RL, Hallcher LM, et al: The effects of lithium on myo-inositol levels in layers of frontal cerebral cortex, in cerebellum, and in corpus callosum of the rat. J Neurochem 34:456–458, 1980

Allsop P, Twigley AJ: The neuroleptic malignant syndrome: case report with a review of the literature. Anaesthesia 42:49–53, 1987

Altshuler LI, Cummings JL, Mills MJ: Mutism: review, differential diagnosis, and report of 22 cases. Am J Psychiatry 143:1409–1414, 1986

Alvord EC, Forno LS: Pathology, in Handbook of Parkinson's Disease. Edited by Koller WC. New York, Marcel Dekker, 1987, pp 209–236

American Psychiatric Association: Diagnostic and Statistical Manual of Mental Disorders, 3rd ed (DSM-III). Washington, DC, American Psychiatric Association, 1980

Ames D, Youl BD: Side effects of Merital (nomifensine). Med J Aust 1:258, 1983

Ananth J, Ruskin R: Unusual reaction to lithium. Can Med Assoc J 111:1049–1050, 1974

Anderson IL, Lipicky RJ, Jones EW: Dantrolene sodium in porcine malignant hyperthermia: studies on isolated muscle strips, in Second International Symposium on

Malignant Hyperthermia. Edited by Aldrete JA, Britt BA. New York, Grune & Stratton, 1978, pp 506–534

Anderson RJ, Reed G, Knochel J: Heatstroke. Adv Intern Med 28:115–140, 1983

Anderson SA, Weinschenk K: Peripheral neuropathy as a component of the neuroleptic malignant syndrome. Am J Med 82:169–170, 1987

Andersson K: Effects of chlorpromazine, imipramine and quinidine on the mechanical activity of single skeletal muscle fibers of the frog. Acta Physiol Scand 85:532–534, 1972

Anden NE, Johnels B: Effects of local application of apromorphine to the corpus striatum and to the nucleus accumbens on the reserpine-induced rigidity in rats. Brain Res 133:386–389, 1977

Ansseau M, Diricq ST, Grisar TH, et al: Biochemical and neuroendocrine approaches to a malignant syndrome of neuroleptics. Acta Psychiatr Belg 80:600–606, 1980

Ansseau M, Reynolds CF, Kupfer DJ, et al: Central dopaminergic and noradrenergic receptor blockade in a patient with neuroleptic malignant syndrome. J Clin Psychiatry 47:320–321, 1986

Appenzeller O, Goss JE: Autonomic deficits in Parkinson's syndrome. Arch Neurol 24:50–57, 1971

Apte SN, Langston JW: Permanent neurological deficits due to lithium toxicity. Ann Neurol 13:453–455, 1983

Araki M, Takagi A, Higuchi I, et al: Neuroleptic malignant syndrome: caffeine contracture of single muscle fibers and muscle pathology. Neurology 38:297–301, 1988

Arana GW, Ornsteen ML, Kanter, et al: The use of benzodiazepines for psychotic disorders: a literature review and preliminary clinical findings. Psychopharmacol Bull 22:77–87, 1986

Armen R, Kanel G, Reynolds T: Phencyclidine-induced malignant hyperthermia causing submassive liver necrosis. Am J Med 77:167–172, 1984

Arnold OH, Stepan H: Untersuchungen zur Frage der akuten tödlichen Katatonie. Wiener Zeitschrift fur Nervenheilkunde und Deren Grenzgebiete 4:235–258, 1952

Aronson MJ, Thompson SV: Complications of acute catatonic excitement: a report of 2 cases. Am J Psychiatry 107:216–220, 1950

Asnis G: Parkinson's disease, depression, and ECT: a review and case study. Am J Psychiatry 134:191–195, 1977

Asnis GM, Asnis D, Dunner DL, et al: Cogwheel rigidity during chronic lithium therapy. Am J Psychiatry 136:1225–1226, 1979

Auzépy PH, Poivet D, Nitenberg G: Insuffisance respiratoire aigue chez deux schizophrenes (rôle éventuel des neuroleptiques retards). La Nouvelle Presse Medicale 6:1236, 1977

Auzépy P, Durocher A, Gay E, et al: Accidents medicamenteux graves chez l'adult: incidents actuelle dans le recrutement des unités de reanimation. La Nouvelle Presse Medicale 8:1315–1318, 1979

Ayd FJ Jr: Fatal hyperpyrexia during chlorpromazine therapy. Journal of Clinical and Experimental Psychopathology 17:189–192, 1956

Ayd FJ Jr: Toxic somatic and psychopathologic reactions to antidepressant drugs. Journal of Neuropsychiatry 2(Suppl 1):119–122, 1961

Ayling JH, Elis FR, Halsall PJ, et al: Thermoregulation and plasma catecholamines during submaximal work in individuals susceptible to malignant hyperpyrexia. Med Sci Sports Exerc 17:274, 1986

Baastrup PC, Hollnagel P, Sorensen R, et al: Adverse reactions in treatment with lithium carbonate and haloperidol. JAMA 236:2645–2646, 1976

Babiak W: Case fatality due to overdosage of a combination of tranylcypromine and imipramine. Can Med Assoc J 85:377, 1961

Badgwell JM, Heavner JE: Masseter spasm heralds malignant

hyperthermia: current dilemma or merely academia gone mad. Anesthesiology 61:230–231, 1984

Baldessarini RJ: Chemotherapy in Psychiatry, 2nd ed. Cambridge, MA, Harvard University Press, 1985

Baldessarini RJ, Stephens JH: Lithium carbonate for affective disorders. Arch Gen Psychiatry 22:72–77, 1970

Baldessarini RJ, Katz B, Cotton P: Dissimilar dosing with high-potency and low-potency neuroleptics. Am J Psychiatry 141:748–752, 1984

Ballard PA, Tetrud JW, Langston JW: Permanent human parkinsonism due to 1-methyl-4-phenyl-1,2,3,6-tetrahydropyridine (MPTP): seven cases. Neurology 35:949–956, 1985

Balster RL: The behavioral pharmacology of phencyclidine, in Psychopharmacology: The Third Generation of Progress. Edited by Meltzer HY. New York, Raven Press, 1987, pp 1573–1578

Balzer H, Hellenbrecht D: Influence of chlorpromazine, prenylamine, imipramine and reserpine on calcium exchange and muscle function. Naunyn Schmiedebergs Arch Pharmacol 264:129–146, 1969

Bamford CB, Bean H: A histological study of a series of cases of acute dementia praecox. Journal of Mental Sciences 78:353–361, 1932

Bark NM: Heatstroke in psychiatric patients: two cases and a review. J Clin Psychiatry 43:377–380, 1982a

Bark NM: The prevention and treatment of heatstroke in psychiatric patients. Hosp Community Psychiatry 33:474–476, 1982b

Barris RW, Schuman HR: Bilateral anterior cingulate gyrus lesions. Neurology (NY) 3:44–52, 1953

Barton CH, Sterling ML, Vaziri ND: Phencyclidine intoxication: clinical experience in 27 cases confirmed by urine assay. Ann Emerg Med 10:243–246, 1981

Bates I, Courtenay-Evans RJ: Neuroleptic malignant syndrome. Br Med J 288:1913, 1984

Behman S: Mutism induced by phenothiazines. Br J Psychiatry 121:599–604, 1972

Beitman BD: Tardive dyskinesia reinduced by lithium carbonate. Am J Psychiatry 135:1229–1230, 1978

Belfer ML, Shader RI: Autonomic effects, in Psychotropic Drug Side Effects: Clinical and Theoretical Perspectives. Edited by Shader RI, DiMascio A. Baltimore, Williams & Wilkins Co, 1970, pp 116–123

Bell LV: On a form of disease resembling some advanced stages of mania and fever. American Journal of Insanity 6:97–127, 1849

Belton NR, Backus RE, Millichap JG: Serum creatine phosphokinase activity in epilepsy. Neurology 17:1073–1076, 1967

Benoit P, Melandri P, Dupont D, et al: Le syndrome malin des neuroleptiques. Concours Med 103:1063–1080, 1981

Bergmann KJ, Limongi JCP, Lowe YH, et al: Potentiation of the "dopa" effect in parkinsonism by a direct GABA receptor agonist. Lancet 1:559, 1984

Bernstein RA: Malignant neuroleptic syndrome: an atypical case. Psychosomatics 20:840–846, 1979

Bernstein WB, Scherokman B: Neuroleptic malignant syndrome in a patient with acquired immunodeficiency syndrome. Acta Neurol Scand 73:636–637, 1986

Bettinger J: Cocaine intoxication: massive oral overdose. Ann Emerg Med 9:429–430, 1980

Biederman J, Lerner Y, Belmaker RH: Combination of lithium carbonate and haloperidol in schizoaffective disorder. Arch Gen Psychiatry 36:327–333, 1979

Billig O, Freeman WT: Fatal catatonia. Am J Psychiatry 100:633–638, 1944

Bismuth C, de Rohan-Chabot P, Goulon M, et al: Dantrolene: a new therapeutic approach to the neuroleptic malignant syndrome. Acta Neurol Scand 70(Suppl 100):193–198, 1984

Blier P, deMontigny C, Chaput Y: Modifications of the serotonin system by antidepressant treatments: implications for the therapeutic response in major depression. J Clin Psychopharmacol 7:245–355, 1987

Bligh J, Cottle WH, Maskrey M: Influence of ambient temperature on the thermoregulatory responses to 5-hydroxytryptamine, noradrenaline and acetylcholine injected into the lateral cerebral ventricles of sheep, goats and rabbits. J Physiol 212:377–392, 1971

Bloom F, Segal D, Ling N, et al: Endorphins: profound behavioral effects in rats suggest new etiological factors in mental illness. Science 194:630–632, 1976

Bloom FE, Baetge G, Deyo S, et al: Chemical and physiological aspects of the actions of lithium and antidepressant drugs. Neuropharmacology 22:359–365, 1983

Blue MG, Schneider SM, Noro S, et al: Successful treatment of neuroleptic malignant syndrome with sodium nitroprusside. Ann Intern Med 104:56–57, 1986

Bohorfoush JG, Craig JB, Patterson HS: Catatonia as a cause of fever of undetermined origin. J Med Assoc Ga 54:324–325, 1965

Boles JM, Lecam B, Mialon P, et al: Hyperthermie maligne des neuroleptiques: guérison rapide par le dantrolene. La Nouvelle Presse Medicale 11:674, 1982

Bond WS: Detection and management of the neuroleptic malignant syndrome. Clin Pharm 3:302–307, 1984

Bond WS, Carvalho M, Foulks EF: Persistent dysarthria with apraxia associated with a combination of lithium carbonate and haloperidol. J Clin Psychiatry 43:256–257, 1983

Borbély AA, Loepfe-Hinkkanen M: Phenothiazines, in Body Temperature: Regulation, Drug Effects, and Therapeutic Implications. Edited by Lomax P, Schönbaum E. New York, Marcel Dekker, 1979, pp 403–426

Borison RL: Amantadine in the management of extrapyramidal side effects. Clin Neuropharmacol 6(Suppl 1):57–63, 1983

Boudduresque G, Poncet M, Ali-Cherif A, et al: Acute encephalopathy during combined phenothiazine and lithium treatment: a new case with low blood lithium. La Nouvelle Presse Medicale 27:2586, 1986

Boulant JA: Hypothalamic control of thermoregulation: neurophysiological basis, in Handbook of the Hypothalamus, Vol 3, Part A. Edited by Morgane PJ, Panksepp J. New York: Marcel Dekker, 1980, pp 1–82

Boulant JA, Demieville HN: Responses of thermosensitive preoptic and septal neurons to hippocampal and brain stem stimulation. J Neurophysiol 40:1356–1368, 1977

Bourgeois M, Tignol J, Henry P: Syndrome malin et morts subites au cours des traitements par neuroleptiques simple et retard. Ann Med Psychol 2:729–746, 1971

Bourgeois M, Tignol J, Villeger M, et al: Le syndrome malin des neuroleptiques: reevaluation a propos de 2 cas. Ann Med Psychol (Paris) 139:547–557, 1981

Bowen LW: Fatal hyperpyrexia with antidepressant drugs. Br Med J 2:1465–1466, 1964

Bowers MB: The role of drugs in the production of schizophreniform psychoses and related disorders, in Psychopharmacology: The Third Generation of Progress. Edited by Meltzer HY. New York, Raven Press, 1987, pp 819–823

Bowman WC, Nott MW: Actions of sympathomimetic amines and their antagonists on skeletal muscle. Pharmacol Rev 21:27–72, 1969

Boyer P: Neuroleptic malignant syndrome: the French data. Presented at the 139th Annual Meeting of the American Psychiatric Association, Washington, DC, May 10–16, 1986

Brachfeld J, Wirtshafter A, Wolfe S: Imipramine-tranylcypromine incompatibility. JAMA 186:1172–1173, 1963

Branchey M, Charles J, Simpson G: Extrapyramidal side effects in lithium maintenance therapy. Am J Psychiatry 133:444–445, 1976

Breakly WR, Kala AK: Typhoid catatonia responsive to ECT. Br Med J 2:357–359, 1977

Brennan D, MacManus M, Howe J, et al: Neuroleptic malignant syndrome without neuroleptics. Br J Psychiatry 152:578–579, 1988

Britt BA: Etiology and pathophysiology of malignant hyperthermia. Fed Proc 38:44–48, 1979

Britt BA, McComas AJ, Endrenyi L, et al: Motor unit counting and the caffeine contracture test in malignant hyperthermia. Anesthesiology 47:490–497, 1977

Brown CS, Wittkowsky AK, Bryant SG: Neuroleptic-induced catatonia after abrupt withdrawal of amantadine during neuroleptic therapy. Pharmacotherapy 6:193–195, 1986

Brown JM: Poisoning with multiple antidepressant drugs. Lancet 1:357, 1970

Brown SJ, Gisolfi CV, Mora F: Temperature regulation and dopaminergic systems in the brain: does the substantia nigra play a role? Brain Res 234:275–286, 1982

Brück K: Heat balance and the regulation of body temperature, in Human Physiology. Edited by Schmidt RF, Thews G. Berlin, Springer-Verlag, 1983, pp 531–547

Brust JC, Hammer JS, Challenor Y, et al: Acute generalized polyneuropathy accompanying lithium poisoning. Ann Neurol 6:360–362, 1979

Buffat JJ, Rouvier PH, Vasseur C, et al: Fallait-il démembrer le syndrome malin des neuroleptiques? Médecine et Armeés 13:767–772, 1985

Bunney BS: Antipsychotic drug effects on the electrical activity of dopaminergic neurons. Trends in Neuroscience 7:212–215, 1984

Bunney WE, Garland-Bunney BL: Mechanisms of action of lithium in affective illness: basic and clinical implications, in Psychopharmacology: The Third Generation of Progress. Edited by Meltzer HY. New York, Raven Press, 1987, pp 553–565

Burch EA, Downs J: Development of neuroleptic malignant syndrome during simultaneous amoxapine treatment and alprazolam discontinuation. J Clin Psychopharmacol 7:55–56, 1987

Burke RE, Fahn S, Mayeux R, et al: Neuroleptic malignant syndrome caused by dopamine-depleting drugs in a patient with Huntington disease. Neurology 31:1022–1026, 1981

Burns RS, Chiueh CC, Markey SP, et al: A primate model of parkinsonism: selective destruction of dopaminergic neurons in the pars compacta of the substantia nigra by N-methyl-4-phenyl-1,2,3,6-tetrahydropyridine. Proc Natl Acad Sci USA 80:4546–4550, 1983

Burns RS, LeWitt PA, Ebert MH, et al: The clinical syndrome of striatal dopamine deficiency. N Engl J Med 312:1418–1421, 1985

Cahill C, Arana GW: Navigating neuroleptic malignant syndrome. Am J Nurs 86:671–673, 1986

Cairns H: Disturbances of consciousness with lesions of the brain-stem and diencephalon. Brain 75:109–146, 1952

Calmeil LF: Dictionnaire de Médecine ou Répertoire Général des Sciences. Médicales sous le Rapport Théorique et Practique (2nd ed). Paris, Béchet, 1832

Campbell IT, Ellis FR, Evans RT: Metabolic rate and blood hormone and metabolite levels of individuals susceptible to malignant hyperpyrexia at rest and in response to food and mild exercise. Anesthesiology 55:46–52, 1981

Campbell IT, Ellis FR, Evans RT, et al: Studies of body temperatures, blood lactate, cortisol and free fatty acid levels during exercise in human subjects susceptible to malignant hyperpyrexia. Acta Anaesthesiol Scand 27:349–355, 1983

Campbell R, Simpson GM: Alternative approaches in the treatment of psychotic agitation. Psychosomatics 27(Suppl):23–27, 1986

Carman JS, Wyatt RJ: Calcium and malignant catatonia. Lancet 2:1124–1125, 1977

Carman JS, Wyatt RJ: Calcium: pacesetting the periodic psychoses. Am J Psychiatry 136:1035–1039, 1979

Carman JS, Wyatt ES, Smith W, et al: Calcium and calcitonin in bipolar affective disorder, in Neurobiology of Mood

Disorders. Edited by Post RM, Ballenger JC. Baltimore, Williams & Wilkins Co, 1984, pp 340–355

Caroff SN: The neuroleptic malignant syndrome. J Clin Psychiatry 41:79–83, 1980

Caroff SN, Mann SC: Neuroleptic malignant syndrome. Psychopharmacol Bull 24:25–29, 1988

Caroff S. Rosenberg H, Hilf M: Dantrolene does not inhibit fluphenazine contractures in-vitro. Pharmacologist 25:130, 1983

Caroff SN, Rosenberg H, Fletcher J, et al: Malignant hyperthermia susceptibility in neuroleptic malignant syndrome. Anesthesiology 67:20–25, 1987a

Caroff SN, Mann SC, Lazarus A: Neuroleptic malignant syndrome. Arch Gen Psychiatry 44:838–839, 1987b

Casey DA: Electroconvulsive therapy in the neuroleptic malignant syndrome. Conv Ther 3:278–283, 1988

Cassidy T, Bansal SK: Neuroleptic malignant syndrome associated with metaclopramide. Br Med J 296:214, 1988

Catravas JD, Waters IW: Acute cocaine intoxication in the conscious dog: studies on the mechanism of lethality. J Pharmacol Exp Ther 217:350–356, 1981

Cavanaugh JJ, Finlayson RE: Rhabdomyolysis due to acute dystonic reaction to antipsychotic drugs. J Clin Psychiatry 45:356–357, 1984

Chavanet P, Portier H, Dumas M: Hyperthermie maligne et rhabdomyolyse fondroyante apres ingestion d'amphetamines. Semaine des Hopitaux de Paris 60:2919–2920, 1984

Chayasirisobhon S, Cullis P, Veeramasuneni RR: Occurrence of neuroleptic malignant syndrome in a narcoleptic patient. Hosp Community Psychiatry 34:548–550, 1983

Cheah KS, Cheah AM: Malignant hyperthermia: molecular defects in membrane permeability. Experientia 41:656–661, 1985

Chesselet MF: Presynaptic regulation of neurotransmitter release in the brain: facts and hypothesis. Neuroscience 12:347–375, 1984

Chiueh CC, Markey SP, Burns RS, et al: Neurochemical and behavioral effects of systemic and intranigral administration of N-methyl-4-phenyl-1,2,3,6-tetrahydropyridine in the rat. Eur J Pharmacol 100:189–194, 1984a

Chiueh CC, Markey SP, Burns RS, et al: Selective neurotoxic effects of N-methyl-4-phenyl-1,2,3,6-tetrahydropyridine (MPTP) in subhuman primates and man: a new animal model of Parkinson's disease. Psychopharmacol Bull 20:548–553, 1984b

Chrisstoffels J, Thiel JH: Delirium acutum, a potentially fatal condition in the psychiatric hospital. Psychiatr Neurol Neurochir 73:177–187, 1970

Ciocatto E, Fagiano G, Bava GL: Clinical features and treatment of overdose of monoamine oxidase inhibitors and their interaction with other psychotropic drugs. Resuscitation 1:69–72, 1972

Clark T, Ananth J, Dubin S: On the early recognition of neuroleptic malignant syndrome. Int J Psychiatry Med 15:299–310, 1986

Clark WG: Changes in body temperature after administration of amino acids, peptides, dopamine, neuroleptics and related agents. Neurosci Biobehav Rev 3:179–231, 1979

Clark WG, Lipton JM: Drug-related heatstroke. Pharmacol Ther 26:345–388, 1984

Clark WG, Lipton JM: Changes in body temperature after administration of adrenergic and serotonergic agents and related drugs including antidepressants II. Neurosci Biobehav Rev 10:153–220, 1986

Claude H, Cuel J: Notes anatomo-cliniques sur trois cas de délire aigu. Encephale 22:628–632, 1927

Clough CG: Neuroleptic malignant syndrome. Br Med J 287:128–129, 1983

Coccaro EF, Siever LJ: Second generation antidepressants: a comparative review. J Clin Pharmacol 25:241–260, 1985

Coffey CE, Ross DR: Treatment of lithium/neuroleptic neurotoxicity during lithium maintenance. Am J Psychiatry 137:736–737, 1980

Coffey CE, Ross DR, Ferren EL, et al: Treatment of the "on-off" phenomenon in parkinsonism with lithium carbonate. Ann Neurol 12:375–379, 1982

Cogen FC, Rigg G, Simmons JL, et al: Phencyclidine-associated acute rhabdomyolysis. Ann Intern Med 88:210–212, 1978

Cohen IM: Complications of chlorpromazine therapy. Am J Psychiatry 113:115–121, 1956

Cohen S, Fligner CL, Raisys VA, et al: A case of nonneuroleptic malignant syndrome. J Clin Psychiatry 48:287–288, 1987

Cohen WJ, Cohen NH: Lithium carbonate, haloperidol, and irreversible brain damage. JAMA 230:1283–1287, 1974

Collins SP, White MD, Denborough MA: The effects of calmodulin antagonist drugs on isolated sarcoplasmic reticulum from malignant hyperpyrexia susceptible swine. Int J Biochem 19:819–826, 1987

Colton CA, Colton JS: The action of dantrolene sodium on the lobster neuromuscular junction. Comp Biochem Physiol 64:153–156, 1979

Condrescu M, Lopez JR, Medina P, et al: Deficient function of the sarcoplasmic reticulum in patients susceptible to malignant hyperthermia. Muscle Nerve 10:238–241, 1987

Conlon P: The spectrum concept of neuroleptic toxicity. Am J Psychiatry 143:811, 1986

Coons DJ, Hillman FJ, Marshall RW: Treatment of neuroleptic malignant syndrome with dantrolene sodium: a case report. Am J Psychiatry 139:944–945, 1982

Corales RL, Maull KI, Becker DP: Phencyclidine abuse mimicking head injury. JAMA 243:2323–2324, 1980

Coryell W, Norby LH, Cohen LH: Psychosis-induced rhabdomyolysis. Lancet 2:381–382, 1978

Cox B: Dopamine, in Body Temperature: Regulation, Drug Effects, and Therapeutic Implications. Edited by Lomax P, Schönbaum E. New York, Marcel Dekker, 1979, pp 231–255

Cox B, Lee TF: Location of receptors mediating hypothermia after injection of dopamine agonists in rats. Br J Pharmacol 59:467–468, 1977

Cox B, Lee TF: Evidence for an endogenous dopamine-mediated hypothermia in the rat. Br J Pharmacol 67:605–610, 1979

Cox B, Lee TF: Further evidence for a physiological role for hypothalamic dopamine in thermoregulation in the rat. J Physiol (Lond) 300:7–17, 1980

Cox B, Tha SJ: The role of dopamine and noradrenaline in temperature control of normal and reserpine-pretreated mice. J Pharm Pharmacol 27:242–247, 1975

Cox B, Kerwin R, Lee TF: Dopamine receptors in the central thermoregulatory pathways of the rat. J Physiol (Lond) 282:471–483, 1978

Cox B, Kerwin RW, Lee TF, et al: A dopamine-5-hydroxytryptamine link in the hypothalamic pathways which mediate heat loss in the rat. J Physiol (Lond) 303:9–21, 1980

Cozzone P, Carrioni P, Desmoulin F, et al: Evolution sous l'effet de la cafeine et de l'ionophone A23187 du pH et des composes phophores intracellulaires du muscle squelettique de porc sensible a l'hyperthermie maligne. Etude en spectroscopie RMN de 31P couplee a l'etude electrophysiologique. J Physiol (Paris) 80:2A, 1985

Cravioto H, Silberman J, Feigin I: A clinical and pathologic study of akinetic mutism. Neurology (NY) 10:10–21, 1960

Creese I, Sibley DR, Hamblin MW, et al: The classification of dopamine receptors: relationship to radioligand binding. Annu Rev Neurosci 6:43–71, 1983

Crews EL, Carpenter AE: Lithium-induced aggravation of tardive dyskinesia. Am J Psychiatry 134:933, 1977

Cruz FG, Thiagarajan D, Harney JH: Neuroleptic malignant syndrome after haloperidol therapy. South Med J 76:684–686, 1983

Cullumbine H, Miles S: The effect of atropine sulphate on men exposed to warm environments. Q J Exp Physiol 41:162–179, 1956

D'Allaire S, DeRoth L: Physiological responses to treadmill exercise and ambient temperature in normal and malignant hyperthermia susceptible pigs. Canadian Journal of Veterinary Research 50:78–83, 1986

Danielson TJ, Coutts RT, Coutts RA, et al: Reserpine induced hypothermia and its reversal by dopamine agonists. Life Sci 37:31–38, 1985

Davidson GM: Concerning the cause of death in certain psychoses. Am J Psychiatry 91:41–49, 1934

Davidson J, McLeod M, Law-Yone B, et al: A comparison of electroconvulsive therapy and combined phenelzine amitriptyline in refractory depression. Arch Gen Psychiatry 35:639–642, 1978

Davies G: Side effects of phenelzine. Br Med J 2:1019, 1960

Davis JM: Antipsychotic drugs, in Comprehensive Textbook of Psychiatry IV, Vol 2. Edited by Kaplan HI, Sadock BJ. Baltimore, Williams & Wilkins Co, 1985, pp 1481–1513

Davis WM, Logston DH, Hickenbottom JP: Antagonism of acute amphetamine intoxication by haloperidol and propranolol. Toxicol Appl Pharmacol 29:397–403, 1974

Delay J, Deniker P: Drug-induced extrapyramidal syndromes, in Handbook of Clinical Neurology, Vol 6: Diseases of the Basal Ganglia. Edited by Vinken PJ, Bruyn GW. Amsterdam, North-Holland, 1968, pp 248–266

Delay J, Pichot P, Lempérière T, et al: Un neuroleptique majeur non phenothiazine et non reserpinique, l'haloperidol, dans le traitement des psychoses. Ann Med Psychol (Paris) 118:145–152, 1960

Delay J, Pichot P, Lempérière T, et al: L'emploi des butyrophenones en psychiatrie: étude statistique et psychometrique, in Symposium Internazionale sull'Haloperidol e Triperidol. Milan, Instituto Luso Farmaco d'Italia, 1962, pp 305–319

Delini-Stula A, Vassout A: Modulation of dopamine-mediated behavioural responses by antidepressants: effects of single and repeated treatment. Eur J Pharmacol 58:443–451, 1979

Demetriou S, Fucek FR, Domino EF: Lack of effect of acute and chronic lithium on chlorpromazine plasma and brain levels in the rat. Common Psychopharmacology 3:17–24, 1979

Denborough MA: Current concepts of the etiology and treatment of malignant hyperthermia, in Second International Symposium on Malignant Hyperthermia. Edited by Aldrete JA, Britt BA. New York, Grune & Stratton, 1978, pp 537–544

Denborough M: Malignant hyperpyrexia. Muscle Nerve 9:30, 1986

Denborough MA, Lovell RRH: Anaesthetic deaths in a family. Lancet 2:45, 1960

Denborough MA, Collins SP, Hopkinson KC: Rhabdomyolysis and malignant hyperpyrexia. Br Med J 288·1878, 1984

Derby IM: Manic-depressive "exhaustive" deaths. Psychiatr Q 7:436–449, 1933

De Roij TAJM, Frens J, Barker J, et al: Thermoregulatory effects of intraventricularly injected dopamine in the goat. Eur J Pharmacol 43:1–7, 1977

De Roij TAJM, Bligh J, Smith CA, et al: Comparison of the thermoregulatory responses to intracerebroventricularly injected dopamine and noradrenaline in the sheep. Naunyn Schmiedebergs Arch Pharmacol 303:263–269, 1978a

De Roij TAJM, Frens J, Woutersen-Van Nijanten F, et al: Comparison of the thermoregulatory responses to intracerebroventricularly injected dopamine, noradrenaline and 5-hydroxytryptamine in the goat. Eur J Pharmacol 49:395–405, 1978b

De Roij TAJM, Frens J, Vianen-Merjerink M, et al: Relation between the thermoregulatory effects of intracerebroventricularly injected dopamine and 5-hydroxytryptamine in the rabbit. Naunyn Schmiedebergs Arch Pharmacol 306:61–66, 1979

Destée A, Lehembre P, Petit H, et al: Encephalopathic toxique par l'association lithium-halopéridol. Lille Médical 23:88–91, 1978

Destée A, Montagne B, Rousseaux M, et al: Incidents et accidents des neuroleptiques (110 hospitalisations en neurologie). Lille Médical 25:291–295, 1980

Devanand DP, Sackeim HA, Finck AD: Modified ECT using succinylcholine after remission of neuroleptic malignant syndrome. Conv Ther 3:284–290, 1988

DeVries DJ, Beart PM: Competitive inhibition of [^{3}H] spiperone binding to D-2 dopamine receptors in striatal homogenates by organic calcium channel antagonists and polyvalent cations. Eur J Pharmacol 106:133–139, 1985

Dhib-Jalbut S, Hesselbrock R, Mouradian MM, et al: Bromocriptine treatment of neuroleptic malignant syndrome. J Clin Psychiatry 48:69–73, 1987

Dilsaver SC: Lithium down-regulates nicotinic receptors in skeletal muscle: cause of lithium-associated myasthenic syndrome? J Clin Psychopharmacol 7:369–370, 1987

Dinarello CA: Pathogenesis of fever, in Cecil Textbook of Medicine (17th ed). Edited by Wyngaarden JB, Smith LH. Philadelphia, WB Saunders Co, 1985, pp 1471–1473

Domino EF: Neurobiology of phencyclidine (sernyl): a drug with an unusual spectrum of pharmacologic activity. International Journal of Neurobiology 6:303–347, 1964

Donaldson IM, Cunningham J: Persisting neurologic sequelae of lithium carbonate therapy. Arch Neurol 40:747–751, 1983

Downey GP, Rosenberg M, Caroff S, et al: Neuroleptic malignant syndrome. Am J Med 77:338–340, 1984

Draper DD, Rothschild MF, Beitz DC, et al: Age and genotype dependent differences in catecholamine concentrations on the porcine caudate nucleus. Exp Gerontol 19:377–381, 1984

Dunn CM, Maltry DE, Eggers GWN: Value of mass spectrometry in early diagnosis of malignant hyperthermia. Anesthesiology 63:333, 1985

Eiser AR, Neff MS, Slifkin RF: Acute myoglobinuric renal failure. Arch Intern Med 142:601–603, 1982

Eles GR, Songer JE, DiPette DJ: Neuroleptic malignant syndrome complicated by disseminated intravascular coagulation. Arch Intern Med 144:1296–1297, 1984

Elizur A, Shopsin B, Gershon S, et al: Intra/extracellular lithium ratios and clinical course in affective states. Clin Pharmacol Ther 13:947–952, 1972

Elizur A, Graff E, Steiner M, et al: Intra/extra red cell lithium and electrolyte distributions as correlates of neurotoxic reactions during lithium therapy, in The Impact of Biology on Modern Psychiatry. Edited by Gershon ES, Belmaker RH, Kety SS, et al. New York, Plenum Press, 1977, pp 55–64

Elliot K, Cole LJ, Frewin DB, et al: Vascular responses in the hands of Parkinson's disease patients. Neurology 24:857–862, 1974

Ellis FR, Halsall PJ: Malignant hyperpyrexia. Br J Hosp Med 24:318–327, 1980

Ellis FR, Halsall PJ: Susceptibility to malignant hyperpyrexia. Anaesthesia 41:85–86, 1986

Ellis FR, Heffron JJA: Clinical and biochemical aspects of malignant hyperpyrexia, in Recent Advances in Anaesthesia and Analgesia. Edited by Atkinson RS, Adams AP. Edinburgh, Churchill Livingstone, 1985, pp 173–207

Ellis KO, Bryant SH: Excitation-contraction uncoupling in skeletal muscle by dantrolene sodium. Naunyn Schmiedebergs Arch Pharmacol 274:107–109, 1972

Ellis KO, Carpenter JF: Studies on the mechanism of action of dantrolene sodium. Naunyn Schmiedebergs Arch Pharmacol 275:83–94, 1972

Ellis KO, Carpenter JF: Mechanism of control of skeletal-muscle contraction by dantrolene sodium. Arch Phys Med Rehabil 55:302–369, 1974

Engel J, Berggren U: Effects of lithium on behavior and central monoamines. Acta Psychiatr Scand 61:133–142, 1980

Eroglu L, Hizal A, Koyuncuogli H: The effect of long-term concurrent administration of chlorpromazine and lithium on the striatal and frontal cortical dopamine metabolism in rats. Psychopharmacology 73:84–86, 1981

European Malignant Hyperpyrexia Group: A protocol for the investigation of malignant hyperpyrexia (MH) susceptibility. Br J Anaesth 56:1267–1269, 1984

Evans DL, Garner BW: Neurotoxicity at therapeutic lithium levels. Am J Psychiatry 136:1481–1482, 1979

Ewert AL, Klock J, Wells B, et al: Neuroleptic malignant syndrome associated with loxapine. J Clin Psychiatry 44:37–38, 1983

Fabre S, Gervais C, Manuel C, et al: Le syndrome malin des neuroleptiques à propos de 7 cas. Encephale 3:321–326, 1977

Fadda F, Serra G, Argiolas A, et al: Effect of lithium on 3, 4-dihydroxy-phenylacetic acid (DOPAC) concentrations in different brain areas of rats. Pharmacol Res Common 12:689–693, 1980

Feibel JH, Schiffer RB: Sympathoadrenomedullary hyperactivity in the neuroleptic malignant syndrome: a case report. Am J Psychiatry 138:1115–1116, 1981

Feigenbaum JJ, Yanai J: Implications of dopamine agonist-induced hypothermia following increased density of dopamine receptors in the mouse. Neuropharmacology 24:735–741, 1985

Fetzer J, Kader G, Danahy S: Lithium encephalopathy: a clinical, psychiatric, and EEG evaluation. Am J Psychiatry 138:1622–1623, 1981

Figa-Talamanca L, Gualandi C, DiMeo L, et al: Hyperthermia after discontinuance of levodopa and bromocriptine therapy: impaired dopamine receptors a possible cause. Neurology 35:258–261, 1985

Finkelman I, Stephens WM: Heat regulation in dementia praecox. Am J Psychiatry 92:1185–1189, 1936

Finlayson RE, Cavanaugh JJ: Drs. Finlayson and Cavanaugh reply (letter). J Clin Psychiatry 45:406, 1985

Finucane P, Murphy SF: Neuroleptic malignant syndrome: common or rare? Ir J Med Sci 13:156, 1984

Fischman MW: Cocaine and the amphetamines, in Psychopharmacology: The Third Generation of Progress. Edited by Meltzer HY. New York, Raven Press, 1987, pp 1543–1553

Fisher KJ, Greiner A: "Acute lethal catatonia" treated by hypothermia. Can Med Assoc J 82:630–634, 1960

Fjalland B: Antagonism of apomorphine-induced hyperthermia in MAOI-pretreated rabbits as a sensitive model of neuroleptic activity. Psychopharmacology 63:119–123, 1979a

Fjalland B: Neuroleptic influence on hyperthermia induced by 5-hydroxy-tryptophan and p-methoxy-amphetamine in MAOI-pretreated rabbits. Psychopharmacology 63:113–117, 1979b

Flemenbaum A: Lithium inhibition of norepinephrine and dopamine receptors. Biol Psychiatry 12:536–572, 1977

Fletcher JE, Rosenberg H: In-vitro interaction between halothane and succinylcholine in human skeletal muscle: implications for malignant hyperthermia and masseter muscle rigidity. Anesthesiology 63:190–194. 1985

Fletcher JE, Rosenberg H, Lizzo F, et al: Strontium and quinacrine antagonize contractures induced by caffeine: implications for malignant hyperthermia. Anesthesiology 65:A238, 1986

Fogel BS, Goldberg RJ: Neuroleptic malignant syndrome. N Engl J Med 313:1292, 1985

Forrest WH: A collaborative clinical trial on trial. Anesthesiology 56:249–250, 1982

Forsman A, Ohman R: Studies on serum protein binding of haloperidol. Curr Ther Res 21:245–255, 1977

Foti ME, Pies RW: Lithium carbonate and tardive dyskinesia. J Clin Psychopharmacol 6:325–326, 1986

Fourrier A: Le syndrome malin existe-t-il encore? Lille Médical 10:404–413, 1965

Frances A, Susman VL: Managing an acutely manic 17-year-old girl with neuroleptic malignant syndrome. Hosp Community Psychiatry 37:771–788, 1986

Franks RD, Aoueille B, Mahowald MC, et al: ECT use for a patient with malignant hyperthermia. Am J Psychiatry 139:1065–1066, 1982

Freeman W, Dumoff E: Cerebellar syndrome following heatstroke. Arch Neurol Psychiatry 51:67–72, 1944

Frey HH: Hyperthermia induced by amphetamine, p-chloroamphetamine and fenfluramine in the rat. Pharmacology 13:163–176, 1975

Fricchione GL: Neuroleptic catatonia and its relationship to psychogenic catatonia. Biol Psychiatry 20:304–313, 1985

Fricchione GL, Cassem NH, Hooberman D, et al: Intravenous lorazepam in neuroleptic-induced catatonia. J Clin Psychopharmacol 3:338–342, 1983

Friedman E, Gershon S: Effect of lithium on brain dopamine. Nature 243:520–521, 1973

Friedman JH, Feinberg SS, Feldman RG: A neuroleptic malignant-like syndrome due to levodopa therapy withdrawal. JAMA 254:2792–2794, 1985

Friedman LS, Weinrauch LA, D'Elia JA: Metoclopramide-induced neuroleptic malignant syndrome. Arch Intern Med 147:1495–1497, 1987

Friedman SA, Hirsch SE: Extreme hyperthermia after LSD ingestion. JAMA 217:1549–1550, 1971

Fuchs F: Thermal inactivation of the calcium regulatory mechanism of human skeletal muscle actomyosin: a possible contributing factor in the rigidity of malignant hyperthermia. Anesthesiology 42:584–589, 1975

Gabris G, Muller C: La catatonie dite "pernicieuse." Encephale 9:365–385, 1983

Gabuzda DH, Frankenburg FR: Fever caused by lithium in a patient with neuroleptic malignant syndrome. J Clin Psychopharmacol 7:283–284, 1987

Gallant EM, Huetteman DA, Donaldson SK: Evidence for excitation-contraction coupling defects in malignant hyperthermia. Muscle Nerve 9:31, 1986

Gallant SM, Godt RE, Gronert GA: Mechanical properties of normal and malignant hyperthermia susceptible porcine muscle: effects of halothane and other drugs. J Pharmacol Exp Ther 213:91–96, 1980

Garbutt JC, van Kammen DP: The interaction between GABA and dopamine: implications for schizophrenia. Schizophr Bull 9:336–353, 1983

Gary NE, Saidi P: Methamphetamine intoxication: a speedy new treatment. Am J Med 64:537–540, 1978

Geisler A, Klysner R: Combined effect of lithium and flupenthixol on striatal adenylate cyclase. Lancet 1:430–431, 1977

Gelenberg AJ: The catatonic syndrome. Lancet 1:1339–1341, 1976

Gelenberg AJ, Mandel MR: Catatonic reactions to high-potency neuroleptic drugs. Arch Gen Psychiatry 34:947–950, 1977

Gelenberg AJ, Bellinghausen B, Wojcik JD, et al: A prospective survey of neuroleptic malignant syndrome in a short-term psychiatric hospital. Am J Psychiatry 145:517–518, 1988

Geller B, Greydanus DE: Haloperidol-induced comatose state with hyperthermia and rigidity in adolescence: two case reports with a literature review. J Clin Psychiatry 40:102–103, 1979

George AL, Wood CA: Succinylcholine-induced hyperkalemia complicating the neuroleptic malignant syndrome. Ann Intern Med 106:172, 1987

Gerlach J, Thorsen K, Munkuud I: Effect of lithium in neuroleptic-induced tardive dyskinesia compared with placebo in a double-blind cross-over trial. Pharmakopsychiatrie Neuropsychopharmakologie 8:51–56, 1975

Gibb WRG: Neuroleptic malignant syndrome in striatonigral degeneration. Br J Psychiatry 153:254–255, 1988

Gibb WRG, Griffith DNW: Levodopa withdrawal syndrome identical to neuroleptic malignant syndrome. Postgrad Med J 62:59–60, 1986

Gibb WRG, Wedzicha JA, Hoffbrand BI: Recurrent neuroleptic malignant syndrome and hyponatremia. J Neurol Neurosurg Psychiatry 49:960–961, 1986

Ginsberg MD, Hertzman M, Schmidt-Nawara WW: Amphetamine intoxication with coagulopathy, hyperthermia, and reversible renal failure. Ann Intern Med 73:81–85, 1970

Giordani L, Amore M, Montanari A, et al: Pridinolum mesylate and neuroleptic malignant syndrome. Am J Psychiatry 142:389–390, 1985

Girke W, Krebs FA, Muller-Oerlinghausen B: Effects of lithium on electromyographic recordings in man. International Pharmacopsychiatry 10:24–36, 1975

Giroud M, Buffat JJ, LeBris H, et al: Insuffisance respiratoire aiguë et traitement psychiatrique au long cours (à propos de onze observations) Lyon Medicine 239:251–255, 1978

Goekoop JG, Carbaat PAT: Treatment of neuroleptic malignant syndrome with dantrolene. Lancet 2:49–50, 1982

Goetz CC, Lutye W, Tanner CM: Autonomic dysfunction in Parkinson's disease. Neurology 36:73–75, 1986

Goldberg LI, Kohli JD, Glock D: Conclusive evidence for two subtypes of peripheral dopamine receptors, in Dopaminergic Systems and Their Regulation. Edited by Woodruff GN, Poat JA, Roberts PJ. Deerfield Beach, FL, VCH Publishers, 1986

Goldney RD, Spence ND: Safety of the combination of

lithium and neuroleptic drugs. Am J Psychiatry 143:882–884, 1986

Golse J, Morel: Delire aigu, neuro-toxicose, syndrome malin et syndrome d'irritation. Encephale 42:422–454, 1953

Gong SNC, Rogers KJ: Role of brain monoamines in the fatal hyperthermia induced by pethidine or imipramine in rabbits pretreated with monoamine oxidase inhibitor. Br J Pharmacol 48:12–18, 1973

Gonzalez MC, Arevalo R, Castro R, et al: Different roles of intra-hypothalamic and nigrostriatal dopaminergic systems in thermoregulatory responses of the rat. Life Sci 39:707–715, 1986

Goodwin GM, Green AR: A behavioural and biochemical study in mice and rats of putative selective agonists and antagonists for $5-HT_2$ and $5-HT_2$ receptors. Br J Pharmacol 84:743–753, 1985

Goodwin GM, DeSouza RJ, Green AR: Presynaptic serotonin receptor-mediated response in mice attenuated by antidepressant drugs and electroconvulsive shock. Nature 317:531–533, 1985

Gorodetzky CW, Isbell H: A comparison of 2,3-dihydrolysergic acid diethylamide with LSD-25. Psychopharmacologia 6:229–233, 1964

Gottlieb JS, Linder S: Body temperature of persons with schizophrenia and of normal subjects. Arch Neurol Psychiatry 33:775–785, 1935

Goulon M, de Rohan-Chabot P, Elkharrat D, et al: Beneficial effects of dantrolene in the treatment of neuroleptic malignant syndrome: a report of two cases. Neurology 33:516–518, 1983

Graham PM, Potter JM, Paterson JW: Combination monoamine oxidase inhibitor/tricyclic antidepressant interaction. Lancet 2:440, 1982

Grahame-Smith DG: Inhibitory effect of chlorpromazine on the syndrome of hyperactivity produced by L-tryptophan or 5-methoxy-N,N-dimethyl-tryptamine in rats treated with a monoamine oxidase inhibitor. Br J Pharmacol 43:856-864, 1971a

Grahame-Smith DG: Studies in-vivo on the relationship between brain tryptophan, brain 5-HT synthesis and hyperactivity in rats treated with a monoamine oxidase inhibitor and L-tryptophan. J Neurochem 18:1053-1066, 1971b

Granato JE, Stern BJ, Ringel A, et al: Neuroleptic malignant syndrome: successful treatment with dantrolene and bromocriptine. Ann Neurol 14:89-90, 1983

Grant R: Neuroleptic malignant syndrome. Br Med J 288:1690, 1984

Green JH, Ellis FR, Halsall PJ, et al: Thermoregulation, plasma catecholamine and metabolite levels during submaximal work in individuals susceptible to malignant hyperpyrexia. Acta Anaesthesiol Scand 31:122-126, 1987

Greenberg LB, Gujavarty K: The neuroleptic malignant syndrome: review and report of three cases. Compr Psychiatry 26:63-70, 1985

Greenberg MS, Gorelick PB: Rigidity and fever in two psychotic patients. Hosp Pract [Off] 21:171-174, 1986

Greenblatt DJ, Gross PL, Harris J, et al: Fatal hyperthermia following haloperidol therapy of sedative-hypnotic withdrawal. J Clin Psychiatry 39:673-675, 1978

Greene DA, Lattimer SA, Sima AAF: Sorbitol, phosophinositides, and sodium-potassium-ATPase in the pathogenesis of diabetic complications. N Engl J Med 316:599-606, 1987

Grey P: Early diagnosis of neuroleptic malignant syndrome. J Clin Psychiatry 47:154, 1986

Grigg JR: Neuroleptic malignant syndrome and malignant hyperthermia. Am J Psychiatry 145:1175, 1988

Grinberg R, Edelist G, Gordon A: Postoperative malignant hyperthermia episodes in patients who received "safe" anaesthetics. Can Anaesth Soc J 30:273-276, 1983

Gronert GA: Contracture responses and energy stores in quadriceps muscle from humans age 7–82 years. Hum Biol 53:43–51, 1980a

Gronert GA: Malignant hyperthermia. Anesthesiology 53:395–423, 1980b

Gronert GA: Controversies in malignant hyperthermia. Anesthesiology 59:273–274, 1983

Gronert GA, Milde JH: Variations in onset of porcine malignant hyperthermia. Anesth Analg 60:499–503, 1981

Gronert GA, Milde JH, Theye RA: Role of sympathetic activity in porcine malignant hyperthermia. Anesthesiology 47:411–415, 1977

Gronert GA, Thompson RL, Onofrio BM: Human malignant hyperthermia: awake episodes and correction by dantrolene. Anesth Analg 59:377–378, 1980

Gronert GA, Ahern CP, Milde JH, et al: Effect of CO_2, calcium, digoxin, and potassium on cardiac and skeletal muscle metabolism in malignant hyperthermia susceptible swine. Anesthesiology 64:24–28, 1986

Gronert GA, Mott J, Lee J: Aetiology of malignant hyperthermia. Br J Anaesth 60:253–267, 1988

Gross P, Hobbs ET, Castronovo FP, et al: Environmental hazards, in MGH Textbook of Emergency Medicine. Edited by Wilkins EW Jr, Dineen JJ, Moncure AC, et al. Baltimore, Williams & Wilkins Co, 1983, pp 177–214

Growe GA, Crayton JW, Klass DB, et al: Lithium in chronic schizophrenia. Am J Psychiatry 136:454–455, 1979

Grunhaus L, Sancovici S, Rimon R: Neuroleptic malignant syndrome due to depot fluphenazine. J Clin Psychiatry 40:99–100, 1979

Gubbay SS, Barwick DD: Two cases of accidental hyperthermia in Parkinson's disease with unusual EEG findings. J Neurol Neurosurg Psychiatry 29:459–466, 1966

Guillemin R: Endorphins, enkephalins and other opioid peptides: their significance in physiology and medicine, in Cecil Textbook of Medicine (17th ed). Edited by

Wyngaarden JB, Smith LH. Philadelphia, WB Saunders Co, 1985, pp 1234–1236

Guyton AC: Textbook of Medical Physiology. Philadelphia, WB Saunders Co, 1986

Häfner H, Kasper S: Akute lebensbedrohliche Katatonie: Epidemiologische und Klinische Befunde. Nervenzart 53:385–394, 1982

Häfner H, Kasper S: Notfall in der Allgemeinmedizin (50): akute lebensbedrohliche Katatonie. Zeitschrift für Alternsforschung (Berlin) 59:665–666, 1983

Haggerty JJ Jr, Bentsen BS, Gillette GM: Neuroleptic malignant syndrome superimposed on tardive dyskinesia. Br J Psychiatry 150:104–105, 1987

Hall GM, Lucke JN: Porcine malignant hyperthermia IX: changes in the concentrations of intramuscular high energy phosphates, glycogen and glycolytic intermediates. Br J Anaesth 55:635–640, 1983

Hall LW, Woolf N, Bradley JWP, et al: Unusual reaction to suxamethonium chloride. Br Med J 2:1305, 1966

Halsall PJ, Ellis FR: The control of muscle contracture by the action of dantrolene on the sarcolemma. Acta Anaesthesiol Scand 27:229–232, 1983

Halsall PJ, Cain PA, Ellis FR: Retrospective analysis of anaesthetics received by patients before susceptibility to malignant hyperpyrexia was recognized. Br J Anaesth 51:949–954, 1979

Hamburg P, Weilburg JB, Cassem NH, et al: Relapse of neuroleptic malignant syndrome with early discontinuation of amantadine therapy. Compr Psychiatry 27:272–275, 1986

Hansen HE, Amdisen A: Lithium intoxication: report of 23 cases and review of 100 cases from the literature. Q J Med 47:123–144, 1978

Hara K, Tohyama I, Kimura H, et al: Reversible serotonergic neurotoxicity of N-methyl-4-pheny-1,2,3,6-tetrahydropyridine (MPTP) in mouse striatum studied by neurochemical and immunohistochemical approaches. Brain Res 410:371–374, 1987

Harriman DGF: Malignant hyperthermia myopathy—a critical review. Br J Anaesth 60:309–316, 1988

Harris M, Nora L, Tanner OM: Neuroleptic malignant syndrome responsive to carbidopa/levodopa: support for a dopaminergic hypothesis. Clin Neuropharmacol 10:186–189, 1987

Harrison GG: Control of malignant hyperthermia syndrome in MHS swine by dantrolene sodium. Br J Anaesth 47:62–65, 1975

Harsch HH: Neuroleptic malignant syndrome: physiological and laboratory findings in a series of nine cases. J Clin Psychiatry 48:328–333, 1987

Hashimoto F, Sherman CB, Jeffery WH: Neuroleptic malignant syndrome and dopaminergic blockade. Arch Intern Med 144:629–630, 1984

Heffron JJA: Sarcolemma, sarcoplasmic reticulum and mitochondria: their relative roles in the pathogenesis of malignant hyperthermia. Muscle Nerve 9:32, 1986

Heikkila RE, Sonsalla PK, Kindt MV, et al: MPTP and animal models of parkinsonism, in Handbook of Parkinson's Disease. Edited by Koller WC. New York, Marcel Dekker, 1987, pp 267–279

Henderson VW, Wooten GF: Neuroleptic malignant syndrome: a pathogenetic role for dopamine receptor blockade? Neurology 31:132–137, 1981

Heninger GR, Charney DS: Mechanism of action of antidepressant treatments: implications for the etiology and treatment of depressive disorders, in Psychopharmacology: The Third Generation of Progress. Edited by Meltzer HY. New York, Raven Press, 1987, pp 535–544

Henry P, Barat M, Bourgeois M: Syndrome malin mortel succédent à une injection d'emblée d'oenanthate de fluphénazine. Presse Med 79:1350, 1971

Hermesh H, Huberman M, Radvan H, et al: Recurrent neuroleptic malignant syndrome due to tiapride and haloperidol: the possible role of D-2 dopamine receptors. J Nerv Ment Dis 172:692–695, 1984

Herzlich BC, Arsura EL, Pagala M, et al: Rhabdomyolysis related to cocaine abuse. Ann Intern Med 109:335–336, 1988

Hesketh JE, Nicolaou NM, Arbuthnott GW, et al: The effect of chronic lithium administration on dopamine metabolism in rat striatum. Psychopharmacology 56:163–166, 1978

Heuser I, Benkert O: Lorazepam for a short-term alleviation of mutism. J Clin Psychopharmacol 6:62, 1986

Hewick DS, Murray N: Red blood cell levels and lithium toxicity. Lancet 2:473, 1976

Hills NF: Combining the antidepressant drugs. Br Med J 1:859, 1965

Himmelhoch JM, Neil JF, May SJ, et al: Age, dementia, dyskinesias and lithium response. Am J Psychiatry 137:941–945, 1980

Himwich WA: Interaction of monoamine oxidase inhibitors with imipramine and similar drugs. Recent Advances in Biological Psychiatry 4:257–268, 1962

Himwich WA, Peterson JC: Effect of the combined administration of imipramine and a monoamine oxidase inhibitor. Am J Psychiatry 117:928–929, 1961a

Himwich WA, Peterson JC: Interaction of imipramine with monoamine oxidase inhibitors. Fed Proc 20:394, 1961b

Hirschorn KA, Greenberg HS: Successful treatment of levodopa-induced myoclonus and levodopa withdrawal-induced neuroleptic malignant syndrome. Clin Neuropharmacology 11:278–281, 1988

Horn E, Lach B, Lapierre Y, et al: Hypothalamic pathology in the neuroleptic malignant syndrome. Am J Psychiatry 145:617–620, 1988

Huber G: Zur nosologischen Differenzierung lebensbedrohlicher katatoner Psychosen. Schweiz Arch Neurol Neurochir Psychiatr 74:216–244, 1954

227

Hughes JR: ECT during and after the neuroleptic malignant syndrome: case report. J Clin Psychiatry 47:42–43, 1986

Ingraham MI, Joo CJ, Tovin K: The neuroleptic malignant syndrome: a case report. Int J Psychiatry Med 12:43–47, 1982

Irwin GE Jr, Simon JE: Neuroleptic malignant syndrome. J Emerg Med 1:207–211, 1984

Ishii T, Sakamoto H, Morimatsu, et al: (A case of cerebral swelling and acute lymphocytic meningitic-encephalitis with clinical symptoms of so-called acute lethal catatonia.) Clin Psychiatry (Tokyo) 14:1043–1047, 1972 (in Japanese)

Itoh H, Ohtsuka N, Ogita K, et al: Malignant neuroleptic syndrome: its present status in Japan and clinical problems. Folia Psychiatr Neurol Jpn 31:565–576, 1977

Izzo KL, Brody R: Rehabilitation in lithium toxicity: case report. Arch Phys Med Rehabil 66:779–782, 1985

Jacobs BL: An animal behavioral model for studying central serotonergic synapses. Life Sci 19:1977, 1976

Jacobs BL, Kleinfuss H: Brainstem and spinal cord mediation of a serotonergic behavioral syndrome. Brain Res 100:450–567, 1975

Jahn D, Greving H: Untersuchung über die körperlichen Störungen bei katatonen Stuporen und der todlichen Katatonie. Archiv fur Psychiatr Nervenkrankh 105:105–120, 1936

James ME: Neuroleptic malignant syndrome in pregnancy. Psychosomatics 29:119–122, 1988

Jan KM, Dorsey S, Bornstein A: Hot hog: hyperthermia from phencyclidine. N Engl J Med 299:722, 1978

Janati A, Webb T: Successful treatment of neuroleptic malignant syndrome with bromocriptine. South Med J 79:1567–1571, 1986

Janowsky EC, Risch C, Janowsky DS: Effects of anesthesia on patients taking psychotropic drugs. J Clin Psychopharm 1:14–20, 1981

Javoy-Agid F, Ruberg M, Pique L: Biochemistry of the hypothalamus in Parkinson's disease. Neurology 34:672–675, 1984

Jefferson JW, Greist JH: Haloperidol and lithium: their combined use and the issue of their compatibility, in Haloperidol Update: 1958–1980. Edited by Ayd FJ Jr. Baltimore, Ayd Medical Communications, 1980, pp 73–82

Jefferson JW, Greist JH, Ackerman DL, et al: Lithium Encyclopedia for Clinical Practice (2nd ed). Washington, DC, American Psychiatric Press, 1987

Jeffries J, Remington G, Wilkins J: The question of lithium/neuroleptic toxicity. Can J Psychiatry 29:601–604, 1984

Jenner P, Marsden CD: Dopamine neurone destruction in human and animal parkinsonism, in Dopaminergic Systems and Their Regulation. Edited by Woodruff GH, Poat JA, Roberts PJ. Deerfield Beach, FL, VCH Publishers, 1986, pp 243–259

Jennings AE, Levey AS, Harrington JT: Amoxapine-associated acute renal failure. Arch Intern Med 143:1525–1527, 1983

Jessee SS, Anderson GF: ECT in the neuroleptic malignant syndrome: case report. J Clin Psychiatry 44:186–188, 1983

Johnels B, Wallin L, Walinder J: Extrapyramidal side effects of lithium treatment. Br Med J 2:642, 1976

Johnson KM: Neurochemistry and neurophysiology of phencyclidine, in Psychopharmacology: The Third Generation of Progress. Edited by Meltzer HY. New York, Raven Press, 1987, pp 1581–1588

Johnson SB, Alvarez WA, Freinhar JP: Rhabdomyolysis in retrospect: psychiatric patients predisposed to this little-known syndrome. Int J Psychiatry Med 17:163–171, 1987

Jones BE, Bobillier P, Pin C, et al: The effect of lesions of catecholamine-containing neurons upon monoamine content of the brain and EEG and behavioral waking in the cat. Brain Res 58:57–177, 1973

Judd FK, Holwill BJ, Normen TR: Liver impairment associated with nomifensine. Aust NZ J Psychiatry 17:288–289, 1983

Juhl RP, Tsuang MT, Perry PJ: Concomitant administration of haloperidol and lithium carbonate in acute mania. Diseases of the Nervous System 38:675–676, 1977

Julien J, Vallat JM, Laguerry A: Myopathy and cerebellar syndrome during acute poisoning with lithium carbonate. Muscle Nerve 2:240, 1979

Jus A, Villaneuve A, Gautier G, et al: Deanol, lithium, and placebo in the treatment of tardive dyskinesia. Neuropsychobiology 4:140–149, 1978

Kalow W, Britt BA, Terreau ME, et al: Metabolic error of muscle metabolism after recovery from malignant hyperthermia. Lancet 2:895–898, 1970

Kane EM, Nutter RW, Weckowicz TE: Response to cutaneous pain in mental hospital patients. J Abnorm Psychol 77:52–60, 1971

Kane J, Rifkin A, Quitkin F, et al: Extrapyramidal side effects with lithium treatment. Am J Psychiatry 135:851–853, 1978

Kaplan RF, Feinglass NG, Webster W, et al: Phenelzine overdose treated with dantrolene sodium. JAMA 255:642–644, 1986

Kaufmann CA, Wyatt RJ: Neuroleptic malignant syndrome, in Psychopharmacology: The Third Generation of Progress. Edited by Meltzer HY. New York, Raven Press, 1987, pp 1421–1430

Keitner GI, Rahman S: Reversible neurotoxicity with combined lithium-haloperidol administration. J Clin Psychopharmacol 4:104–105, 1984

Kelemen J, Slonim A, Hubay M, et al: Ambulatory malignant hyperthermia syndrome: successful treatment with dantrolene sodium. Neurology 36:240, 1986

Kelkar VV, Doctor RB, Jindal MN: Chlorpromazine-induced contracture of frog rectus abdominis muscle. Pharmacology 12:32–38, 1974

Keller HH, Schaffner R, Haefely W: Interaction of benzodiazepines with neuroleptics at central dopamine neurons. Naunyn Schmiedebergs Arch Pharmacol 294:1–7, 1976

Keltner NL, McIntyre CW: Neuroleptic malignant syndrome. J Neurosurg Nurs 17:362–366, 1985

Kendrick WC, Hull AR, Knochel JP: Rhabdomyolysis and shock after intravenous amphetamine administration. Ann Intern Med 86:381–387, 1977

Kerr DD, Wingard DW, Gatz EE: Prevention of porcine malignant hyperthermia by oral dantrolene, in Second International Symposium on Malignant Hyperthermia. Edited by Aldrete JA, Britt BA. New York, Grune & Stratton, 1978, pp 499–507

Kick K: Fieberzustande unter psychopharmakotherapie: differencialtypologie und diagnostik. Pharmakopsychiatrie 14:12–20, 1981

Kilbourne EM, Choi K, Jones TS, et al: Risk factors for heatstroke: a case-control study. JAMA 247:3332–3336, 1982

Kim J, Hassler R: Effect of acute haloperidol on the gamma-aminobutyric acid system in rat striatum and substantia nigra. Brain Res 88:150–153, 1975

Kimsey LR, Gibbs JT, Glen RS, et al: The neuroleptic malignant syndrome. Tex Med 79:54–55, 1983

Kinross-Wright VJ: Trifluoperazine and schizophrenia, in Trifluoperazine: Clinical and Pharmacologic Aspects. Edited by Brill H. Philadelphia, Lea & Febiger, 1958, pp 62–70

Kirkpatrick B, Edelsohn GA: Risk factors for the neuroleptic malignant syndrome. Psychiatric Medicine 2:371–381, 1985

Kiyohara T, Hori T, Shibata M, et al: Neuronal inputs to preoptic thermosensitive neurons: histological and electrophysiological mapping of central connections. Journal of Thermal Biology 9:21–26, 1984

Klein SK, Levinsohn MW, Blumer JL: Accidental chlorpromazine ingestion as a cause of neuroleptic malignant syndrome in children. J Pediatr 107:970–973, 1985

Klip A, Britt BA, Elliot ME, et al: Changes in cytoplasmic free calcium caused by halothane. Role of the plasma membrane and intracellular Ca^{2+} stores. Biochem Cell Biol 64:1181–1189, 1986

Klock JC, Boerner U, Becker EE: Coma, hyperthermia, and bleeding associated with massive LSD overdose. West J Med 120:183–188, 1973

Knochel JP: Clinical physiology of heat exposure, in Disorders of Fluid and Electrolyte Metabolism. Edited by Maxwell MH, Kluman CR. New York, McGraw-Hill, 1980

Knochel JP: Rhabdomyolysis and myoglobinuria, in The Kidney in Systemic Disease. Edited by Suki W, Eknoyan G. New York, John Wiley & Sons, 1981, pp 263–284

Knochel JP: Disorders due to heat and cold, in Cecil Textbook of Medicine (17th ed). Edited by Wyngaarden JB, Smith LH, Philadelphia, WB Saunders Co, 1985, pp 2304–2307

Knoll H: Clinical-genealogical contribution to the problem of pernicious catatonia (English translation). Archiv fur Psychiatr Nervenkrantz 192:1–33, 1954

Kojima I, Kojima K, Krentler D, et al: The temporal integration of the aldosterone secretory response to angiotensin occurs via two intracellular pathways. J Biol Chem 259:14448–14457, 1984

Kolb ME, Horne ML, Martz R: Dantrolene in human malignant hyperthermia: a multi-center study. Anaesthesiology 56:254–262, 1982

Kollias J, Bullard RW: The influence of chlorpromazine on physical and chemical mechanism of temperature regulation in the rat. J Pharmacol Exp Ther 145:373–381, 1964

Konikoff F, Kuritzky A, Jerushalmi Y, et al: Neuroleptic malignant syndrome induced by a single injection of haloperidol. Br Med J 289:1228–1229, 1984

Kontaxakis V, Stefanis C, Markidis M, et al: Neuroleptic malignant syndrome in a patient with Wilson's disease. J Neurol Neurosurg Psychiatry 51:1001–1002, 1988

Kopin IJ: Neurotoxins affecting biogenic aminergic neurons, in Psychopharmacology: The Third Generation of Progress. Edited by Meltzer HY. New York, Raven Press, 1987, pp 351–358

Kosten TR, Kleber HD: Sudden death in cocaine abusers: relation to neuroleptic malignant syndrome. Lancet 1:1198–1199, 1987

Kosten TR, Kleber HD: Rapid death during cocaine abuse: a variant of the neuroleptic malignant syndrome? Am J Drug Alcohol Abuse 14:335–346, 1988

Koziel-Schminda E: "Ostra Smierteina Katatonia" Typu Staudera O Przebiegu Letalnym (Analiza Materialow Kliniczynch I Sekcyjnch Szpitala W Kochborowie Z Lat 1950–1970). Psychiatr Pol 7:563–567, 1973

Kraepelin E: Lectures on Clinical Psychiatry (2nd ed). Edited by Johnstone T. New York, William Wood, 1905

Kraines SH: Bell's mania (acute delirium). Am J Psychiatry 91:29–40, 1934

Krishna NR, Taylor MA, Abrams R: Combined haloperidol and lithium carbonate in treating manic patients. Compr Psychiatry 19:119–120, 1978

Krisko I, Lewis E, Johnson JE: Severe hyperpyrexia due to tranylcypromine-amphetamine toxicity. Ann Intern Med 70:559–564, 1969

Krivosic-Horber R, Adnet P, Guevart E, et al: Neuroleptic malignant syndrome and malignant hyperthermia. Br J Anaesth 59:1554–1556, 1987

Krohn KD, Slowman-Kovacs S, Leapman SB: Cocaine and rhabdomyolysis. Ann Intern Med 108:639–640, 1988

Krull F, Risse A: Neuroleptic malignant syndrome with

rhabdomyolysis and therapy with physostigmine. Fortschr Neurol Psychiatr 54:398–401, 1986

Kuehnle JC: Strategies in treatment of psychosis in remission. Unpublished paper presented at Psychiatric Grand Rounds, Temple University Health Sciences Center, Philadelphia, Pennsylvania, October 7, 1983

Kuhn WF, Lippmann SB: Neuroleptic malignant syndrome as a possible postoperative complication: case report. Gen Hosp Psychiatry 9:179–181, 1987

Kuncl RW, Meltzer HY: Pathologic effect of phencyclidine and restraint on rat skeletal muscle: prevention by prior denervation. Exp Neurol 45:387–402, 1974

Kurlan R, Hamill R, Shoulson I: Neuroleptic malignant syndrome. Clin Neuropharmacol 7:109–120, 1984

Ladame C: Psychose aiguë idiopathique ou foudroyante. Schweizer Archiv fur Neurologic und Psychiatrie 5:3–28, 1919

Lader M: Combined use of tricyclic antidepressants and monoamine oxidase inhibitors. J Clin Psychiatry 44:20–24, 1983

Lagarde P, Reis J, Hemmendinger S, et al: Le syndrome malin des neuroleptiques est-il comparable a l'hyperthermie maligne par anesthesie? Presse Med 15:1376–1377, 1986

Lal S, Nair NPV, Guyda H: Effect of lithium on hypothalamic-pituitary dopaminergic function. Acta Psychiatr Scand 57:91–96, 1978

Lang A: Dopamine agonists in the treatment of dystonia. Clin Neuropharmacol 8:38–57, 1985

Langston JW, Forno LS: The hypothalamus in Parkinson disease. Ann Neurol 3:129–133, 1978

Langston JW, Langston EB, Irwin I: MPTP-induced parkinsonism in human and non-human primates: clinical and experimental aspects. Acta Neurol Scand 70(Suppl 100):49–54, 1984

Larach MG, Rosenberg H, Larach DR, et al: Prediction of malignant hyperthermia susceptibility by clinical signs. Anesthesiology 66:547–550, 1987

Larson CP: Fatal cases of acute manic-depressive psychosis. Am J Psychiatry 95:971–982, 1939

Laskowska D, Chrzanowicz T: Proba Leczenia Trifluoperazyna (Stelazyna) Ostrych Stanow Amentywno-Katatonicznych Psychozy Schizofrenicznej. Psychiatr Pol 3:681–684, 1967

Laskowska D, Urbaniak K, Jus A: The relationship between catatonia-delirious states and schizophrenia in the light of a follow-up study (Stauder's lethal catatonia). Br J Psychiatry 111:254–257, 1965

Lavie CJ, Olmsted TR, Ventura HO, et al: Neuroleptic malignant syndrome: an underdiagnosed reaction to neuroleptic agents? Postgrad Med 80:171–178, 1986a

Lavie CJ, Ventura HO, Walker G: Neuroleptic malignant syndrome: three episodes with different drugs. South Med J 79:1571–1573, 1986b

Lazarus A: Heatstroke in a chronic schizophrenic patient treated with high-potency neuroleptics. Gen Hosp Psychiatry 7:361–363, 1985a

Lazarus A: Neuroleptic malignant syndrome and amantadine withdrawal. Am J Psychiatry 142:142, 1985b

Lazarus A: Neuroleptic malignant syndrome: detection and management. Psychiatr Ann 15:706–712, 1985c

Lazarus A: Psychiatric patients at high risk for rhabdomyolysis. J Clin Psychiatry 45:406, 1985d

Lazarus A: Therapy of neuroleptic malignant syndrome. Psychiatr Dev 1:19–30, 1986a

Lazarus A: Treatment of neuroleptic malignant syndrome with electroconvulsive therapy. J Nerv Ment Dis 174:47–49, 1986b

Lazarus AL, Toglia JU: Fatal myoglobinuric renal failure in a patient with tardive dyskinesia. Neurology 35:1055–1057, 1985

Lebensohn ZM, Jenkins RB: Improvement of parkinsonism in depressed patients treated with ECT. Am J Psychiatry 132:283–285, 1975

Lee FI: Imipramine overdosage: report of a fatal case. Br Med J 1:338–339, 1961

Lee TF, Mora F, Myers RD: Dopamine and thermoregulation: an evaluation with special reference to dopaminergic pathways. Neurosci Biobehav Rev 9:589–598, 1985

Lees H: The effects of 1-(1-phenyl cyclohexyl) piperidine hydrochloride (sernyl) on rat liver mitochondria. Neuropharmacol 20:306, 1961

Lefkowitz D, Ford CS, Rich C, et al: Cerebellar syndrome following neuroleptic induced heatstroke. J Neurol Neurosurg Psychiatry 46:183–185, 1983

Lesaca T: Amoxapine and neuroleptic malignant syndrome. Am J Psychiatry 144:1514, 1987

Lesser MS, Kahan M, Brenner R, et al: Dantrolene sodium as a possible prophylactic agent against NMS. Hillside J Clin Psychiatry 8:34–37, 1986

Levenson JL: Neuroleptic malignant syndrome. Am J Psychiatry 142:1137–1145, 1985

Levenson JL: Diagnosing and treating neuroleptic malignant syndrome (reply). Am J Psychiatry 143:675, 1986

Levenson JL, Fisher JG: Long-term outcome after neuroleptic malignant syndrome. J Clin Psychiatry 49:154–156, 1988

Levinson DF, Simpson GM: Neuroleptic-induced extrapyramidal symptoms with fever: heterogeneity of the "neuroleptic malignant syndrome." Arch Gen Psychiatry 43:839–848, 1986

Lew TY, Tollefson G: Chlorpromazine-induced neuroleptic malignant syndrome and its response to diazepam. Biol Psychiatry 18:1441–1446, 1983

Lewis DA: Unrecognized chronic lithium neurotoxic reactions. JAMA 250:2029–2030, 1983

Lewis E: Hyperpyrexia with antidepressant drugs. Br Med J 1:1671, 1965

Liden CB, Lovejoy FH, Costello CE: Phencyclidine: nine cases of poisoning. JAMA 234:513–516, 1975

Lieberman A, Gopinathan G: Treatment of "on-off" phenomena with lithium. Ann Neurol 12:402, 1982

Lieberman JA, Kane JM, Reife R: Neurotransmitter effects of monoamine oxidase inhibitors. J Clin Psychopharmacol 5:221–228, 1985

Lieberman JA, Kane JM, Reife R: Neuromuscular effects of monoamine oxidase inhibitors. Adv Neurol 43:231–249, 1986

Lin KM, Pollard RE, Lesser IM: Ethnicity and psychopharmacology. Cult Med Psychiatry 10:151–165, 1986

Lin MT, Wang HC, Chandra A: The effects on thermoregulation of intracerebroventricular injection of acetylcholine, pilocarpine, physostigmine, atropine and hemicholinium in the rat. Neuropharmacology 18:561–565, 1980

Linden CH, Rumack BH, Strehlke C: Monoamine oxidase inhibitor overdose. Ann Emerg Med 13:1137–1144, 1984

Lindesay J: Neuroleptic malignant syndrome and lethal catatonia. Br J Psychiatry 148:342–343, 1986

Lindvall O, Björklund A, Skagerberg G: Dopamine-containing neurons in the spinal cord: anatomy and some functional aspects. Ann Neurol 14:255–260, 1983

Lindvall O, Björklund A: Neuroanatomy of central dopamine pathways: review of recent progress, in Advances in the Biosciences, vol 37: Advances in Dopamine Research. Edited by Kohosaka M, Shohomori T, Tsukada Y, et al. Oxford, Pergamon, 1982, pp 297–311

Lingjaerde O: Contributions to the study of schizophrenia and the acute, malignant deliria. J Oslo City Hosp 14:43–83, 1963

Linnoila M, Karoum F, Rosenthal N, et al: Electroconvulsive treatment and lithium carbonate: their effects on norephinephrine metabolism in patients with primary major depressions. Arch Gen Psychiatry 40:677–680, 1983

Litovitz TL, Troutman WG: Amoxapine overdose: seizures and fatalities. JAMA 250:1069–1071, 1983

Loghmanee F, Tobak M: Fatal malignant hyperthermia

associated with recreational cocaine and ethanol abuse. Am J Forensic Med Pathol 7:246–248, 1986

Login IS, Cronin MJ, MacLeod RM: Neuroleptic malignant syndrome caused by dopamine depleting drugs. Neurology 32:218-219, 1982

Lopez JR, Alamo L, Caputo C, et al: Intracellular ionized calcium concentration in muscles from humans with malignant hyperthermia. Muscle Nerve 8:355–358, 1985

Lopez JR, Medina P, Alamo L: Dantrolene sodium is able to reduce the resting ionic (Ca^{2+}) in muscle from humans with malignant hyperthermia. Muscle Nerve 10:77–79, 1987

Lotstra F, Linkowski P, Mendlewicz J: General anesthesia after neuroleptic malignant syndrome. Biol Psychiatry 18:243–247, 1983

Loudon JB, Waring H: Toxic reactions to lithium and haloperidol. Lancet 2:1088, 1976

Loveless AH, Maxwell DR: A comparison of the effects of imipramine, trimipramine and some other drugs in rabbits treated with a monoamine oxidase inhibitor. Br J Pharmacol 25:158–170, 1965

Lowance D: Heat injury: a possible association with lithium carbonate therapy. J Med Assoc Ga 69:284–286, 1980

Lucke JN, Hall GM, Lister D: Malignant hyperthermia and the role of stress. Ann NY Acad Sci 317:336–337, 1979

Lutsky I, Witkowski J, Henschel EO: HLA typing in a family prone to malignant hyperthermia. Anesthesiology 56:224–226, 1982

Lutz EG: Neuroleptic-induced akathisia and dystonia triggered by alcohol. JAMA 236:2422–2423, 1976

Lydiatt JS, Hill GE: Treatment of heatstroke with dantrolene. JAMA 246:41–42, 1981

Maggi A, Enna SJ: Regional alterations in rat brain neurotransmitter systems following chronic lithium treatment. J Neurochem 34:888–892, 1980

Maickel RP: Interaction of drugs with autonomic nervous

function and thermoregulation. Fed Proc 29:1973–1979, 1970

Maitre A, Boucharlat J, Vincent T, et al: La catatonie aiguë léthale: considerations cliniques, psychopathologiques et préventives. Ann Med Psychol (Paris) 140:1149–1154, 1982

Malamud N, Boyd DA: Sudden "brain death" in schizophrenia with extensive lesions in the cerebral cortex. Arch Neurol Psychiatry 41:352–364, 1939

Malamud N, Haymaker W, Custer RP: Heatstroke: a clinico-pathologic study of 125 fatal cases. Military Surgeon 99:397–449, 1946

Mann SC, Boger WP: Psychotropic drugs, summer heat and humidity, and hyperpyrexia: a danger restated. Am J Psychiatry 135:1097–1100, 1978

Mann SC, Caroff SN: Lethal catatonia and the neuroleptic malignant syndrome. Am J Psychiatry 144:1106–1107, 1987

Mann SC, Greenstein RA: Hyperpyrexia related to neuroleptic treatment. Scientific Proceedings of the American Psychiatric Association 136:227, 1983

Mann SC, Greenstein RA, Eilers R: Early onset of severe dyskinesia following lithium-haloperidol treatment. Am J Psychiatry 140:1385–1386, 1983

Mann SC, Caroff SN, Bleier HR, et al: Lethal catatonia. Am J Psychiatry 143:1374–1381, 1986

Marjanen LA, Collins SP, Denborough MA: Calmodulin and malignant hyperpyrexia. Biochem Med 32:283–287, 1984

Marley E, Wozniak KM: Clinical and experimental aspects of interactions between amine oxidase inhibitors and amine re-uptake inhibitors. Psychol Med 13:735–749, 1983

Marra JP, Minta DL, Hobbins TE: Suicide by the ingestion of tranylcypromine. JAMA 192:1104–1105, 1965

Marsden CD, Jenner P: The pathophysiology of extrapyramidal side-effects of neuroleptic drugs. Psychol Med 10:55–72, 1980

Martin ML, Lucid EJ, Walker RW: Neuroleptic malignant syndrome. Ann Emerg Med 14:354–358, 1985

May DC, Morris SW, Stewart RM, et al: Neuroleptic malignant syndrome: response to dantrolene sodium. Ann Intern Med 98:183–184, 1983

May RH: Catatonic-like states following phenothiazine therapy. Am J Psychiatry 115:1119–1120, 1959

Mazzia VDB, Simon A: Medicolegal implications of malignant hyperpyrexia, in Second International Symposium on Malignant Hyperthermia. Edited by Aldrete JA, Britt BA. New York, Grune & Stratton, 1978, pp 545–551

McCarron MM, Schulze BW, Thompson GA, et al: Acute phencyclidine intoxication: clinical patterns, complications, and treatment. Ann Emerg Med 10:290–297, 1981a

McCarron MM, Schulze BW, Thompson GA, et al: Acute phencyclidine intoxication: incidence of clinical findings in 1000 cases. Ann Emerg Med 10:237–242, 1981b

McCarthy A, Bourke S, Fahy J, et al: Fatal recurrence of neuroleptic malignant syndrome. Br J Psychiatry 152:558–559, 1988

McCurdy RL, Kane FJ: Transient brain syndrome as a non-fatal reaction to combined pargyline-imipramine treatment. Am J Psychiatry 121:397–398, 1964

McEvoy JP: Rapid shifts in therapeutic and extrapyramidal effects of neuroleptics. Am J Psychiatry 143:1504, 1986

McEvoy JP, Lohr JB: Diazepam for catatonia. Am J Psychiatry 141:284–285, 1984

McGrath CJ, Lee JC, Rempel WE: Halothane testing for malignant hyperthermia in swine: dose-response effects. Am J Vet Res 45:1734–1736, 1984

McPherson E, Taylor CA: The genetics of malignant hyperthermia: evidence for heterogeneity. Am J Med Genet 11:273–385, 1982

Meller E, Friedman E: Lithium dissociates haloperidol-induced behavioral supersensitivity from reduced DOPAC increase in rat striatum. Eur J Pharmacol 76:25–29, 1981

Meltzer HY: Rigidity, hyperpyrexia and coma following fluphenazine enanthate. Psychopharmacologia 29:337–346, 1973

Meltzer HY, Holtzman PS, Hassu SJ, et al: Effect of phencyclidine and stress on plasma creatine phosphokinase (CPK) and aldolase activity in man. Psychopharmacologia 26:44–53, 1972

Meltzer HY, Ross-Stanton J, Schlessinger S: Mean serum creatine kinase activity in patients with functional psychoses. Arch Gen Psychiatry 37:650–655, 1980

Menes C, Burra P, Hoaken PCS: Untoward effects following combined neuroleptic-lithium therapy: cardiac arrhythmics and seizure. Can J Psychiatry 25:573–576, 1980

Menon MK, Vivonia CA: Modification of apomorphine hypothermia by drugs affecting brain 5-hydroxytryptamine function. Eur J Pharmacol 76:223–227, 1981

Mereu G, Fanni B, Gessa GL: General anesthetics prevent dopaminergic neuron stimulation by neuroleptics, in Catecholamines: Neuropharmacology and Central Nervous System–Theoretical Aspects. Edited by Usdin E, Dahlström A, Engel J. New York, Alan R. Liss, 1984, pp 353–358

Merigian KS, Roberts JR: Cocaine intoxication: hyperpyrexia, rhabdomyolysis and acute renal failure. Clinical Toxicology 25:135–148, 1987

Merriam AE: Neuroleptic malignant syndrome after imipramine withdrawal. J Clin Psychopharmacol 7:53–54, 1987

Merry SN, Werry JS, Merry AF, et al: The neuroleptic malignant syndrome in an adolescent. J Am Acad Child Psychiatry 25:284–286, 1986

Meyers EF, Meyers RW: Thermic stress syndrome. JAMA 247:2098–2099, 1982

Mickelson JR, Ross JA, Reed BK, et al: Enhanced Ca^{2+}-induced calcium release by isolated sarcoplasmic reticulum vesicles from malignant hyperthermia susceptible pig muscle. Biochim Biophys Acta 862:318–328, 1986

Mickelson JR, Ross JA, Hyslop RJ, et al: Skeletal muscle sarcolemma in malignant hyperthermia: evidence for a defect in calcium regulation. Biochim Biophys Acta 897:364–376, 1987

Miller F, Menninger J: Correlation of neuroleptic dose and neurotoxicity in patients given lithium and a neuroleptic. Hosp Community Psychiatry 38:1219–1221, 1987a

Miller F, Menninger J: Lithium-neuroleptic neurotoxicity is dose dependent. J Clin Psychopharmacol 7:89–91, 1987b

Miller F, Menninger J, Whitcup SM: Lithium-neuroleptic neurotoxicity in the elderly bipolar patient. J Clin Psychopharmacol 6:176–178, 1986

Mirchandani H, Reich LE: Fatal hyperthermia as a result of ingestion of tranylcypromine combined with white wine and cheese. J Forensic Sci 30:217–220, 1985

Misiaszek JJ, Potter RL: Atypical neuroleptic malignant syndrome responsive to conservative management. Psychosomatics 26:62–66, 1985

Miyoshi K, Tadeo D, Susumi H, et al: (Febrile episodes and catatonia). Psychiatr Neurol Jpn 70:52–65, 1968 (in Japanese)

Modigh K, Balldin J, Eriksson E, et al: Increased responsiveness of dopamine receptors after ECT: a review of experimental and clinical evidence, in ECT: Basic Mechanisms. Edited by Lerer B, Weiner RD, Belmaker RH. Washington, DC, American Psychiatric Press, 1986

Molokov AN: (On acute delirium syndrome in periodic catatonia and in infections). Zh Nevropatol Psikhiatr 62:866–873, 1962 (in Russian)

Moore A, O'Donohoe NV, Monaghan H: Neuroleptic malignant syndrome. Arch Dis Child 61:793–795, 1986

Moore KE: Hypothalamic dopaminergic neuronal systems, in Psychopharmacology: The Third Generation of Progress. Edited by Meltzer HY. New York, Raven Press, 1987, pp 127–139

Morant JCA: A catatonic syndrome resulting in death. Can J Psychiatry 29:147–150, 1984

Morris HH, McCormick WF, Reinarz JA: Neuroleptic malignant syndrome. Arch Neurol 37:462–463, 1980

Moulds RFW, Denborough MA: Biochemical basis of malignant hyperpyrexia. Br Med J 2:241–244, 1974

Moyes DG: Malignant hyperpyrexia caused by trimeprazine. Br J Anaesth 45:1163–1164, 1973

Mueller EA, Murphy DL, Sunderland T: Further studies of the putative serotonin agonist, m-chlorophenylpiperazine: evidence for a serotonin receptor mediated mechanism of action in humans. Psychopharmacology 89:388–391, 1986

Mueller PS: Neuroleptic malignant syndrome. Psychosomatics 26:654–662, 1985

Mueller PS, Vester JW, Fermaglich J: Neuroleptic malignant syndrome: successful treatment with bromocriptine. JAMA 249:386–388, 1983

Myers RD: Hypothalamic control of thermoregulation: neurochemical mechanisms, in Handbook of the Hypothalamus, Vol 3, Part A. Edited by Morgane PJ, Panksepp J. New York, Marcel Dekker, 1980, pp 83–210

Myers RD, Waller MB: Thermoregulation and serotonin, in Serotonin in Health and Disease, Vol 2. Edited by Essman WB. New York, Spectrum Publications, 1978, pp 1–67

Neil JF, Himmelhoch JM, Licata SM: Emergence of myasthenia gravis during treatment with lithium carbonate. Arch Gen Psychiatry 33:1090–1092, 1976

Nelson TE, Chausmer AB: Calcium content and contracture in isolated muscle of malignant hyperthermia in pigs. J Pharmacol Exp Ther 219:107–111, 1981

Nelson TE, Denborough MA: Studies on normal human skeletal muscle in relation to the pathopharmacology of malignant hyperpyrexia. Clin Exp Pharmacol Physiol 4:315–322, 1977

Nelson TE, Flewellen EH: Rationale for dantrolene vs. procainamide for treatment of malignant hyperthermia. Anesthesiology 50:118–122, 1979

Nelson TE, Flewellen EH: The malignant hyperthermia syndrome. N Engl J Med 309:416–418, 1983

Nelson TE, Bedell DM, Jones EW: Porcine malignant hyperthermia: effects of temperature and extracellular calcium concentration on halothane-induced contracture of susceptible skeletal muscle. Anesthesiology 42:301–306, 1975

Nelson TE, Austin KL, Denborough MA: Screening for malignant hyperpyrexia. Br J Anaesth 29:169–171, 1977

Nelson TE, Flewellen EH, Arnett DW: Prolonged electromechanical coupling time intervals in skeletal muscle of pigs susceptible to malignant hyperthermia. Muscle Nerve 6:263–268, 1983

Nelson TE, Belt HW, Kennamer DL, et al: Studies on the Ca^{2+} transport function of sarcoplasmic reticulum isolated from human malignant hyperthermia skeletal muscle. Anesthesiology 65:A243, 1986

Nelson TE, Flewellen EH, Belt MW, et al: Calcium and magnesium content of skeletal muscle: studies in subjects undergoing diagnostic testing for malignant hyperthermia. Br J Anaesth 59:730–734, 1987a

Nelson TE, Flewellen EH, Belt MW, et al: Comparison of Ca^{++} uptake and spontaneous Ca^{++} release from sarcoplasmic reticulum vesicles isolated from muscle of malignant hyperthermia diagnostic patients. J Pharmacol Exp Ther 240:785–788, 1987b

Nemes ZC, Volavka J, Lajtha A, et al: Concurrent lithium administration results in higher haloperidol levels in brain and plasma of guinea pigs. Psychiatry Res 20:313–316, 1987

Nesemann ME, Michels JT, Pollei SR: Neuroleptic malignant syndrome. Wis Med J 83:12–14, 1984

Nestelbaum Z, Siris SG, Rifkin A, et al: Exacerbation of

schizophrenia associated with amantadine. Am J Psychiatry 143:1170–1171, 1986

Nestoros JN, Nair NPV, Pulman JR, et al: High doses of diazepam improve neuroleptic-resistant chronic schizophrenic patients. Psychopharmacology 81:42–47, 1983

Neubauer KR, Kaufman RD: Another use for mass spectrometry: detection and monitoring of malignant hyperthermia. Anesth Analg 64:837–839, 1985

Neveu P, Marrel P, Marchandon AM, et al: Catatonie maligne: traitement par hibernation. Ann Med Psychol (Paris) 131:267–274, 1973

Newman PK, Saunders M: Lithium neurotoxicity. Postgrad Med J 55:701–703, 1979

Newmann MA: Periventricular diffuse pinealoma: report of a case with clinical features of catatonic schizophrenia. J Nerv Ment Dis 121:193–204, 1955

Norman AB, Wylie GL, Prince AK: Supersensitivity of d-amphetamine-induced hyperthermia in rats following continuous treatment with neuroleptics. Eur J Pharmacol 140:349–351, 1987

O'Brien PJ: Porcine malignant hyperthermia susceptibility: hypersensitive calcium release mechanism of skeletal muscle sarcoplasmic reticulum. Canadian Journal of Veterinary Research 50:318–328, 1986a

O'Brien PJ: Porcine malignant hyperthermia susceptibility: increased calcium-sequestering activity of skeletal muscle sarcoplasmic reticulum. Canadian Journal of Veterinary Research 50:329–337, 1986b

Oefele KV, Grohmann R, Ruther E: Adverse drug reactions in combined tricyclic and MAOI therapy. Pharmacopsychiatry 19:243–244, 1986

Ohnishi ST, Waring AJ, Fang SRG, et al: Abnormal membrane properties of the sarcoplasmic reticulum of pigs susceptible to malignant hyperthermia: modes of action of halothane, caffeine, dantrolene and two other drugs. Arch Biochem Biophys 247:294–301, 1986

Oikkonen M, Rosenberg PH, Bjorkenheim JM: Spinal block, after dantrolene pretreatment for resection of a thigh muscle herniation in a young malignant hyperthermia susceptible man. Acta Anaesthesiol Scand 31:309–311, 1987

Oku S, Liew CC, Britt BA: Analysis of sarcoplasmic reticulum poteins in patients susceptible to malignant hyperthermia. J Neurol Sci 60:127–135, 1983

Okumura F, Crocker BD, Denborough MA: Identification of susceptibility to malignant hyperpyrexia in swine. Br J Anaesth 51:171–176, 1979

Olgin J, Argov Z, Rosenberg H, et al: Non-invasive evaluation of malignant hyperthermia susceptibility with phosphorus nuclear magnetic resonance spectroscopy. Anesthesiology 68:507–513, 1988

Olson KR, Benowitz NL: Life-threatening cocaine intoxication. Problems in Critical Care 1:95–105, 1987

Ording H: Incidence of malignant hyperthermia in Denmark. Anesth Analg 64:700–704, 1985

Ording H: Diagnosis of susceptibility to malignant hyperthermia in man. Br J Anaesth 60:287–302, 1988

Ording H, Nielsen VG: Atracurium and its antagonism by neostigmine (plus glycopyrrotate) in patients susceptible to malignant hyperthermia. Br J Anaesth 58:1001–1004, 1986

Ording H, Skovgaard LT: In vitro diagnosis of susceptibility to malignant hyperthermia: comparison between dynamic and static halothane and caffeine tests. Acta Anaesthesiol Scand 31:458–461, 1987

Ording H, Ranklev E, Fletcher R: Investigation of malignant hyperthermia in Denmark and Sweden. Br J Anaesth 56:1183–1190, 1984

Ording H, Hald A, Sjontoft E: Malignant hyperthermia triggered by heating in anaesthetized pigs. Acta Anaesth Scand 29:698–701, 1985

Ostrow DG, Sontham AS, Davis JM: Lithium-drug interactions altering the intracellular lithium level: an in-vitro study. Biol Psychiatry 15:723–739, 1980

Paasuke RT: Drugs, heat stroke and dantrolene. Can Med Assoc J 130:341–343, 1984

Paasuke RT, Brownell AKW: Amide local anaesthetics and malignant hyperthermia. Canadian Anaesthesiology Society Journal 33:126–129, 1986a

Paasuke RT, Brownell AKW: Serum creatine kinase level as a screening test for susceptibility to malignant hyperthermia. JAMA 255:769–711, 1986b

Page P, Morgan M, Loh L: Ketamine anesthesia in pediatric procedures. Acta Anaesth Scand 16:155–160, 1972

Palmer H: Potentiation of pethidine. Br Med J 2:944, 1960

Pandey GN, Goel I, Davis JM: Effect of neuroleptic drugs on lithium uptake for the human erythrocyte. Clin Pharmacol Ther 26:96–102, 1979

Papez JW: A proposed mechanism of emotion. Arch Neurol Psychiatry 38:725–741, 1937

Parini M, Archambeaud-Mouveroux F, Vincent D, et al: Association d'une crise aigue thyrotoxique et d'un syndrome malin des neuroleptiques efficacie de la bromocriptine. Presse Med 13:1902, 1984

Patel P, Bristow G: Postoperative neuroleptic malignant syndrome: a case report. Can J Anaesth 34:515–518, 1987

Patterson JF: Neuroleptic malignant syndrome associated with metoclopramide. South Med J 81:674–675, 1988

Patti F, Maccagnano C, Panico AM, et al: Effects of dantrolene sodium on GABAergic activity in spinal cord, corpus striatum, substantia nigra and cerebral cortex in rat. Acta Neurol (Napoli) 36:384–388, 1981

Pearlman CA: Neuroleptic malignant syndrome: a review of the literature. J Clin Psychopharmacol 6:257–273, 1986

Peebles-Brown AE: Hyperpyrexia following psychotropic drug overdose. Anaesthesia 40:1097–1099, 1985

Pelonero AL, Levenson JL, Silverman JJ: Neuroleptic therapy following neuroleptic malignant syndrome. Psychosomatics 26:946–948, 1985

Penn H, Racy J, Lapham L, et al: Catatonic behavior, viral encephalopathy and death. Arch Gen Psychiatry 27:758–761, 1972

Penney JB, Young AB: Speculations on the functional anatomy of basal ganglia disorders. Annu Rev Neurosci 6:73–94, 1984

Pert A, Rosenblatt JE, Sivit C, et al: Long term treatment with lithium prevents the development of dopamine receptor supersensitivity. Science 201:171–173, 1978

Pestronk A, Drachman DB: Lithium reduces the number of acetylcholine receptors in skeletal muscle. Science 210:342–343, 1980

Petersdorf RG: Alterations in body temperature, in Harrison's Principles of Internal Medicine (8th ed). Edited by Thorn GW, Adams RD, Braunwald E, et al. New York, McGraw-Hall, 1977, pp 53–59

Pfeiffer RF, Sucha EL: On-off induced malignant hyperthermia. Ann Neurol 18:138–139, 1985

Pirovino M, Meier J, Meyer M, et al: Malignant neuroleptic-like syndrome (English translation). Dtsch Med Wochenschr 109:378–381, 1984

Pittman KJ, Jakubavic A, Febiger HC: The effects of chronic lithium on behavioral and biochemical indices of dopamine receptor supersensitivity in the rat. Psychopharmacology 82:371–377, 1984

Pope HG Jr, Jonas JM, Hudson JI, et al: Toxic reactions to the combination of monoamine oxidase inhibitors and tryptophan. Am J Psychiatry 142:491–492, 1985

Pope HG Jr, Cole JO, Choras PT, et al: Apparent neuroleptic malignant syndrome with clozapine and lithium. J Nerv Ment Dis 174:493–495, 1986a

Pope HG Jr, Keck PE Jr, McElroy SL: Frequency and presentation of neuroleptic malignant syndrome in a large psychiatric hospital. Am J Psychiatry 143:1227–1233, 1986b

Powers P, Douglass TS, Waziri R: Hyperpyrexia in catatonic states. Diseases of the Nervous System 37:359–361, 1976

Prakash R, Kelwala S, Ban TA: Neurotoxicity in patients treated for schizophrenia during lithium therapy. Compr Psychiatry 23:271–273, 1982a

Prakash R, Kelwala S, Ban TA: Neurotoxicity with combined administration of lithium and a neuroleptic. Compr Psychiatry 23:567–571, 1982b

Preston J: Central nervous system reactions to small doses of tranquilizers. Am Prac Dig Tr 10:627–630, 1959

Price WA, Giannini AJ: A paradoxical response to chlorpromazine: a possible variant of the neuroleptic malignant syndrome. J Clin Pharmacol 23:567–569, 1983

Price WA, Zimmer B, Kucas P: Serotonin syndrome: a case report. J Clin Pharmacol 26:77–78, 1986

Primeau F, Fontaine R, Chouinard G: Poorly controlled EPS: risk factors for NMS. Can J Psychiatry 32:238–329, 1987

Prunier PG, Frankel BL: Atypical fatal hyperpyrexia: a case report. J Clin Psychopharmacol 6:322–323, 1986

Przewlocka B, Kaluza J: The effect of intraventricularly administered noradrenaline and dopamine on the body temperature of the rat. Pol J Pharmacol Pharm 25:345–355, 1973

Puech AJ, Chermat R, Poncelet M, et al: Antagonism of hypothermia and behavioral response to apomorphine: a simple, rapid and discriminating test for screening antidepressants and neuroleptics. Psychopharmacology 75:84–91, 1981

Pumariega AJ, Muller B, Rivers-Bulkeley N: Acute renal failure secondary to amoxapine overdose. JAMA 248:3141–3142, 1982

Putney JW, Bianchi CP: Site of action of dantrolene in frog sartorius muscle. J Pharmacol Exp Ther 189:202–217, 1974

Quinn NP: Levodopa, in Handbook of Parkinson's Disease. Edited by Koller WC. New York, Marcel Dekker, 1987, pp 317–337

Ranklev E, Fletcher R, Krantz P: Malignant hyperpyrexia and sudden death. Am J Forensic Med Pathol 6:149–150, 1985

Ranklev E, Fletcher R, Blomquist S: Static v. dynamic tests in the in vitro diagnosis of malignant hyperthermia susceptibility. Br J Anaesth 58:646–648, 1986

Rappolt RJ, Gay GR, Farris RD: Emergency management of acute phencyclidine intoxication. Journal of the American College of Emergency Physicians 8:68–76, 1979

Rasmussen H: The calcium messenger system I. N Engl J Med 314:1094–1100, 1986a

Rasmussen H: The calcium messenger system II. N Engl J Med 314:1164-1170, 1986b

Ravi SD, Borge GF, Roach FL, et al: Neuroleptics, laryngeal-pharyngeal dystonia, and acute renal failure. J Clin Psychiatry 43:300, 1982

Razani J, White KL, White J, et al: The safety and efficacy of combined amitriptyline and tranylcypromine antidepressant treatment: a controlled trial. Arch Gen Psychiatry 40:657–661, 1983

Reches A, Fahn S: Lithium in the "on-off" phenomenon. Ann Neurol 14:91–92, 1983

Reches A, Wagner HR, Jackson V, et al: Chronic lithium administration has no effect on haloperidol induced supersensitivity of pre- and postsynaptic dopamine receptors in rat brain. Brain Res 246:172–177, 1982

Reches A, Jackson-Lewis V, Fahn S: Lithium does not interact with haloperidol in the dopaminergic pathways of the rat brain. Psychopharmacology 82:330–334, 1984

Reda FA, Escobar JI, Scanlow JM: Lithium carbonate in the treatment of tardive dyskinesia. Am J Psychiatry 132:560–562, 1975

Redalié L: Contribution à l'étude de l'anatomie pathologique du délire aigu idiopathique. Schweizer Archiv fur Neurologie und Psychiatric 7:35, 1920

Regestein QR, Alpert JS, Reich P: Sudden catatonic stupor with disastrous outcome. JAMA 238:618–620, 1977

Reis J, Felten P, Rumbach L, et al: Hyperthermie avec rhabdomyolyse aigue chez un psychotique traite par neuroleptiques. Rev Neurol (Paris) 139:595–596, 1983

Renshaw PF, Summers JJ, Renshaw CE, et al: Changes in the ^{31}P-NMR spectra of cats receiving lithium chloride systemically. Biol Psychiatry 21:694–698, 1986a

Renshaw PF, Joseph NE, Leigh JS: Chronic dietary lithium induces increased levels of myo-inositol-1-phosphatase activity in rat cerebral cortex homogenates. Brain Res 380:401–404, 1986b

Richards GA, Fritz VU, Pincus P, et al: Unusual drug interactions between monoamine oxidase inhibitors and tricyclic antidepressants. J Neurol Neurosurg Psychiatry 50:1240–1241, 1987

Richter MA, Joffe RT: Use of tricyclic antidepressants in a patient with malignant hyperthermia. Am J Psychiatry 144:526, 1987

Ries RK, Schuckit MA: Catatonia and autonomic hyperactivity. Psychosomatics 21:349–350, 1980

Rifkin A, Quitkin F, Klein DF: Organic brain syndrome during lithium carbonate therapy. Compr Psychiatry 14:251–254, 1973

Ritchie P: Neuroleptic malignant syndrome. Br Med J 287:560–561, 1983

Rivera-Calimlin L, Kerzner B, Karch FE: Effect of lithium on plasma chlorpromazine levels. Clin Pharmacol Ther 23:451–455, 1978

Robbins TW, Everitt BJ: Functional studies of the central catecholamines. Int Rev Neurobiol 23:303–365, 1982

Roberts AN: The value of ECT in delirium. Br J Psychiatry 109:653–655, 1963

Roberts JR, Quattrocchi E, Howland MA: Severe hyperthermia secondary to intravenous drug abuse. Am J Emerg Med 2:373, 1984

Robertson JC: Recovery after massive monoamine oxidase inhibitor overdose complicated by malignant hyperpyrexia treated with chlorpromazine. Postgrad Med J 48:64–65, 1972

Robinson MB, Kennett RP, Harding AE, et al: Neuroleptic malignant syndrome associated with metoclopramide. J Neurosurg Psychiatry 40:1304–1312, 1985

Rock E, Kozak-Reiss G: Effect of halothane on the Ca^{2+} transport system of surface membranes isolated from normal and malignant hyperthermia pig skeletal muscle. Arch Biochem Biophys 256:703–707, 1987

Roervik S, Stovner J: Ketamine-induced acidosis, fever and creatine kinase rise. Lancet 2:1384–1385, 1974

Rogers JD, Stoudemire GA: Neuroleptic malignant syndrome in multiple sclerosis: possible masking effects of antispasmodics. Psychosomatics 29:221–223, 1988

Rogers KJ: Role of brain monoamines in the interaction between pethidine and tranylcypromine. Eur J Pharmacol 14:86–88, 1971

Rogers KJ, Thornton JA: The interaction between monoamine oxidase inhibitors and narcotic analgesics in mice. British Journal of Pharmacology and Chemotherapy 36:470–480, 1969

Rosenberg H: Sites and mechanism of action of halothane on skeletal muscle function in vitro. Anesthesiology 50:331–335, 1979

Rosenberg H, Fletcher JE: Masseter muscle rigidity and malignant hyperthermia susceptibility. Anesth Analg 65:161–164, 1986

Rosenberg H, Fletcher JE: Malignant hyperthermia, in Muscle Relaxants: Side Effects and a Rational Approach to Selection. Edited by Azar I. New York, Marcel Dekker, 1987, pp 115–148

Rosenberg H, Reed S: In-vitro contracture test for susceptibility to malignant hyperthermia. Anesth Analg 62:415–420, 1983

Rosenblatt JE, Pert A, Layton B, et al: Chronic lithium reduces [^{3}H]-spiroperidol binding in rat striatum. Eur J Pharmacol 67:321–322, 1980

Ross ED, Stewart RM: Akinetic mutism from hypothalamic damage: successful treatment with dopaminergic agonists. Neurology (NY) 31:1435–1439, 1981

Ross-Canada J, Chizzonite RA, Meltzer HY: Retention of sarcoplasmic calcium inhibits development of the phencyclidine-restraint experimental myopathy. Exp Neurol 79:1–10, 1983

Rosse R, Ciolino C: Dopamine agonists and neuroleptic malignant syndrome. Am J Psychiatry 142:270–271, 1985

Roszell DK, Horita A: The effects of haloperidol and thioridazine on apomorphine- and LSD-induced hyperthermia in the rabbit. J Psychiatr Res 12:117–123, 1975

Roth D, Alarcón FJ, Fernandez JA, et al: Acute rhabdomyolysis associated with cocaine intoxication. N Engl J Med 319:673–677, 1988

Roth RH, Wolf ME, Deutsch AY: Neurochemistry of midbrain dopamine systems, in Psychopharmacology: The Third Generation of Progress. Edited by Meltzer HY, New York, Raven Press, 1987, pp 81–94

Roth SD, Addonizio G, Susman VL: Diagnosing and treating neuroleptic malignant syndrome. Am J Psychiatry 143:673, 1986

Rothke S, Bush D: Neuropsychological sequelae of neuroleptic malignant syndrome. Biol Psychiatry 21:838–841, 1986

Rupniak NHJ, Jenner P, Marsden CD: Acute dystonia induced by neuroleptic drugs. Psychopharmacology 88:403–419, 1986

Russell VA, Nurse B, Lamm MCL, et al: Effect of chronic antidepressant treatment on noradrenergic modulation of ^{3}H-dopamine release from rat nucleus accumbens and striatal slices. Brain Res 410:78–82, 1987

Rutberg H, Hakanson E, Hall GM, et al: Effects of graded exercise on leg exchange of energy substrates in malignant hyperthermia susceptible subjects. Anesthesiology 65:A239, 1986

Ruwe WD, Myers RD. Dopamine in the hypothalamus of the cat: pharmacological characterization and push-pull perfusion analysis of sites mediating hypothermia. Pharmacol Biochem Behav 9:65–80, 1978

Sachdev PS: Lithium potentiation of neuroleptic-related extrapyramidal side effects. Am J Psychiatry 143:942, 1986

Sackeim HA, Decina P, Prohovnik I, et al: Anticonvulsant and antidepressant properties of electroconvulsive therapy: a proposed mechanism of action. Biol Psychiatry 18:1301–1310, 1983

Salam SA, Pillai AK, Beresford TP: Lorazepam for psychogenic catatonia. Am J Psychiatry 144:1082–1083, 1987

Samie MR: Neuroleptic malignant-like syndrome induced by metoclopramide. Movement Disorders 2:57–60, 1987

Sandyk R: The endogenous opioid system in neurological disorders of the basal ganglia. Life Sci 37:1655–1663, 1985a

Sandyk R: Neuroleptic malignant syndrome and the opioid system. Med Hypotheses 17:133–138, 1985b

Sandyk R, Hurwitz MD: Toxic irreversible encephalopathy induced by lithium carbonate and haloperidol. S Afr Med J 64:875–876, 1983

Sangal R, Dimitrijevic R: Neuroleptic malignant syndrome. JAMA 254:2795–2796, 1985

Sansone MEG, Ziegler DK: Lithium neurotoxicity: a review of neuroleptic complications. Clin Neuropharmacol 8:242–248, 1985

Satinoff E: Neural organization and evolution of thermal regulation in mammals. Science 201:16–22, 1978

Scarlett JD, Zimmerman R, Berkovic SF: Neuroleptic malignant syndrome. Aust NZ J Med 13:70–73, 1983

Scatton B, Rouquier L, Javoy-Agid F, et al: Dopamine deficiency in the cerebral cortex in Parkinson's disease. Neurology 32:1039–1040, 1982

Scheid KF: Die Somatopathologie der Schizophrenie. Zeitschrift fur die Gesamte Neurol und Psychiatrie 163:585–603, 1938

Scheideggar W: Katatone Todesfälle in der Psychiatrischen Klinik von Zurich con 1900 bis 1928. Zeitschrift fur die Gesamte Neurol und Psychiatrie 120:587–649, 1929

Schibuk M, Schachter D: A role for catecholamines in the pathogenesis of neuroleptic malignant syndrome. Can J Psychiatry 31:66–69, 1986

Schilder P: Psychic disturbances after head injuries. Am J Psychiatry 91:155–188, 1934

Schmauss M, Kapfhammer HP, Meyr P, et al: Combined MAO-inhibitor and tri(tetra)-cyclic antidepressant treatment in therapy resistant depression: a retrospective study. Pharmacopsychiatry 19:251–252, 1986

Schmidt RM, Zacher G: Bedrohliche Katatonie: Entität oder multigenetisches Syndrome? Übersicht und Untersuchung an 50 Fällen. Psychiatr Clin (Basel) 7:65–74, 1974

Schou M: Long-lasting neurological sequelae after lithium intoxication. Acta Psychiatr Scand 70:594–602, 1984

Schou M, Amdisen A, Trap-Jensen J: Lithium poisoning. Am J Psychiatry 125:520–527, 1968

Schrader GD: Neuroleptic malignant syndrome. Med J Aust 69:367, 1982

Schulte-Sasse U, Komar K, Eberlein HJ: Dantrolen in der Behandlung lebensbedrohlicher psychiatrischer Krankheitsbilder. Dtsch Med Wochenschr 110:457–461, 1985

Schultz W: The role of the primate nigrostriatal dopamine system in the initiation and conduction of behavioral acts, as derived from single cell recordings and MPTP induced lesion effects, in Neurotransmitter Interactions in the Basal Ganglia. Edited by Sandler M, Feuerstein C, Scatton B. New York, Raven Press, 1987, pp 95–100

Schuster CR, Lewis M, Seiden LS: Fenfluramine neurotoxicity. Psychopharmacol Bull 22:148–151, 1986

Schvehla TS, Herjanic M: Neuroleptic malignant syndrome, bromocriptine, and anticholinergic drugs. J Clin Psychiatry 49:283–284, 1988

Schwartz JG, McAfee RD: Cocaine and rhabdomyolysis. J Fam Pract 24:209, 1987

Schwartz L, Rockoff MA, Koka BU: Masseter spasm with anesthesia: incidence and implications. Anesthesiology 61:772, 1984

Scott NR, Boulant JA: Dopamine effects on thermosensitive neurons in hypothalamic tissue slices. Brain Res 306:157–163, 1984

Sechi GP, Tanda F, Mutani R: Fatal hyperpyrexia after withdrawal of levodopa. Neurology 34:249–251, 1984

Sedivic V: (Psychoses endangering life). Cesk Psychiatr 77:38–41, 1981 (in Czech)

Seiden LS, Ricaurte GA: Neurotoxicity of methamphetamine and related drugs, in Psychopharmacology: The Third Generation of Progress. Edited by Meltzer HY. New York, Raven Press, 1987, pp 359–366

Sellers EM, Roy ML, Martin PR, et al: Amphetamines, in Body Temperature: Regulation, Drug Effects and Therapeutic Implications. Edited by Lomax P, Schonbaum E. New York, Marcel Dekker, 1979, pp 461–498

Sellers J, Tyler P, Whitley A, et al: Neurotoxic effects of lithium with delayed rise in serum lithium levels. Br J Psychiatry 140:623–625, 1982

Selye H: The Stress of Life. New York, McGraw-Hill, 1956

Shader RI, Greenblatt DJ: Uses and toxicity of belladonna alkaloids and synthetic anticholinergics. Seminars in Psychiatry 3:449–476, 1971

Shalev A, Munitz H: The neuroleptic malignant syndrome: agent and host interaction. Acta Psychiatr Scand 73:337–347, 1986

Shalev A, Aizenberg D, Hermesh H, et al: Summer heat and

the neuroleptic malignant syndrome (English translation). Harefuah 110:6–8, 1986

Shalev A, Hermesh H, Munitz H: The role of external heat load in triggering the neuroleptic malignant syndrome. Am J Psychiatry 145:110–111, 1988

Sherman CB, Hashimoto F, Davidson EJ: Gas-producing Escherichia coli fasciitis in a patient with the neuroleptic malignant syndrome. JAMA 250:361, 1983

Sherman WR, Munsell LY, Gish BG, et al: Effects of systemically administered lithium on phosphoinositide metabolism in rat brain, kidney and testis. J Neurochem 44:798–807, 1985

Shibolet S, Lancaster MC, Danyon Y: Heat stroke: a review. Aviat Space Environ Med 47:280–301, 1976

Shields WD, Bray PF: A danger of haloperidol therapy in children. J Pediatr 88:301–303, 1976

Shimomura K, Hashimoto M, Mori J, et al: Role of brain amines in the fatal hyperpyrexia caused by tranylcypromine in LiCl-pretreated rats. Jpn J Pharmacol 29:161–170, 1979

Shopsin B, Gershon S: Cogwheel rigidity related to lithium maintenance. Am J Psychiatry 132:536–538, 1975

Shopsin B, Johnson G, Gershon S: Neurotoxicity with lithium: differential drug responsiveness. Int Pharmacopsychiatry 5:170, 1970

Shopsin B, Small JG, Kellaus JJ, et al: Combining lithium and neuroleptics. Am J Psychiatry 133:980–981, 1976

Shulack NR: Sudden "exhaustive" death in excited patients. Psychiatr Q 18:3–12, 1944

Shulack NR: Exhaustion syndrome in excited psychotic patients. Am J Psychiatry 102:466–475, 1946

Sieber FE, McShane AJ: Neuroleptic malignant syndrome. N Engl J Med 313:1292, 1985

Simpson DL, Rumack BH: Methylene dioxyamphetamine: clinical description of overdose, death and review of pharmacology. Arch Intern Med 141:1507–1509, 1981

Simpson DM, Davis GC: Case report of neuroleptic malignant syndrome associated with withdrawal from amantadine. Am J Psychiatry 141:796–797, 1984

Simpson GK, Davidson NM: Possible hepatotoxicity of zimelidine. Br Med J 287:1181, 1983

Simpson GM, Branchey MH, Lee JH, et al: Lithium in tardive dyskinesia. Pharmacopsychiatry 9:76–80, 1976

Singh G: The malignant neuroleptic syndrome (a review with report of three cases). Indian Journal of Psychiatry 23:179–183, 1981

Singh H: Atropine-like poisoning due to tranquilizing agents. Am J Psychiatry 117:360–361, 1960

Singh SV: Lithium carbonate/fluphenazine decanoate producing irreversible brain damage. Lancet 2:278, 1982

Singh TH: Neuroleptic malignant syndrome. Br J Psychiatry 145:98, 1984

Small JG, Kellams JJ, Milstein V, et al: A placebo-controlled study of lithium combined with neuroleptics in chronic schizophrenic patients. Am J Psychiatry 132:1315–1317, 1975

Smith DF, Shimizu M, Schon M: Lithium absorption, distribution and clearance and body temperature in rats given lithium plus haloperidol. Pharmacology 15:337–340, 1977

Smith RE, Helms PM: Adverse effects of lithium therapy in the acutely ill elderly patient. J Clin Psychiatry 43:94–99, 1982

Smith RJ, Newbegin HF, Ellis FR: Anxiety, hypothalamic-pituitary-adrenal axis activity and malignant hyperpyrexia. Psychopharmacology 89:S33, 1986

Smithson WA, Gronert GA, Moss KK: Dantrolene and potentially fatal hyperthermia secondary to L-asparaginase. Cancer Treat Rep 67:318–319, 1983

Snider RM, Fisher SK, Agranoff BW: Inositide-linked second messengers in the central nervous system, in Psychopharmacology: The Third Generation of Progress. Edited by Meltzer HY. Raven Press, New York, 1987, pp 317–324

Snyder SH, Greenberg D, Yamamara HI: Antischizophrenic drugs and brain cholinergic receptors. Arch Gen Psychiatry 31:58–61, 1974

Somers CJ, McLoughlin JV: Malignant hyperthermia in pigs: calcium ion uptake by mitochondria from skeletal muscle in susceptible animals given neuroleptic drugs and halothane. J Comp Pathol 92:191–195, 1982

Sonnenklar N, Rendell-Baker L: Hyperpyrexia during pregnancy. Lancet 2:43, 1972

Souliere CR, Weintraub SJ, Kirchner JC: Markedly delayed postoperative malignant hyperthermia. Archives of Otolaryngology, Head, and Neck Surgery 112:564–566, 1986

Sours JA: Akinetic mutism simulating catatonic schizophrenia. Am J Psychiatry 119:451–455, 1962

Spring GK: EEG observations in confirming neurotoxicity. Am J Psychiatry 136:1099–1100, 1979a

Spring GK: Neurotoxocity with combined use of lithium and thioridazine. J Clin Psychiatry 40:135–138, 1979b

Spring G, Frankel M: New data on lithium and haloperidol incompatibility. Am J Psychiatry 138:245–252, 1981

Standish-Barry HMAS, Shell MA: Toxic neurological reaction to lithium/thioridazine. Lancet 1:771, 1983

Stanec A, Stefano G: Cyclic AMP in normal and malignant hyperpyrexia susceptible individuals following exercise. Br J Anaesth 56:1243–1246, 1984

Starr MS, Summerhayes M, Kilpatrick IC: Interactions between dopamine and gamma-aminobutyrate in the substantia nigra: implications for the striatonigral output hypothesis. Neuroscience 8:547–559, 1983

Stauder KH: Die tödliche Katatonie. Archiv fur Psychiatr Nervenkrantz 102:614–634, 1934

Staunton DA, Magistretti PJ, Schoemaker WJ, et al: Effects of chronic lithium treatment on dopamine receptors in the rat corpus striatum, I: locomotor activity and behavioral supersensitivity. Brain Res 232:391–400, 1982a

Staunton DA, Magistretti PJ, Schoemaker WJ, et al: Effects of chronic lithium treatment on dopamine receptors in the rat corpus striatum, II: no effect on denervation or neuroleptic-induced supersensitivity. Brain Res 232:401–412, 1982b

Steele TE: Adverse reactions suggesting amoxapine-induced dopamine blockade. Am J Psychiatry 139:1500–1501, 1982

Stefanini E, Lougori R, Fadda F, et al: Inhibition by lithium of dopamine-sensitive adenylate cyclase in the rat brain. J Neurochem 30:257–258, 1978

Stitt JT: Fever versus hyperthermia. Fed Proc 38:39–43, 1979

Stoudemire A, Luther JS: Neuroleptic malignant syndrome and neuroleptic-induced catatonia: differential diagnosis and treatment. Int J Psychiatry Med 14:57–63, 1984

Straker M: Neuroleptic malignant syndrome: fatalities associated with neuroleptic use and schizophrenia. Psychiatr J Univ Ottawa 11:28–30, 1986

Strayhorn JM, Nash JL: Severe neurotoxicity despite "therapeutic" serum lithium levels. Diseases of the Nervous System 38:107–111, 1977

Sukanova L: Maligni neuroleptiky syndrom. Ceskoslovenska Psychiatrie 81:91–95, 1985

Sulpizio A, Fowler PJ, Macko E: Antagonism of fenfluramine-induced hyperthermia: a measure of central serotonin inhibition. Life Sci 22:1439–1446, 1978

Suranyi-Cadotte BE, Nestoros JN, Nair NPV, et al: Parkinsonism induced by high doses of diazepam. Biol Psychiatry 20:451–460, 1985

Surmont DWA: Coma in a young woman: a case of malignant hyperthermia. Tijdschr Geneeskunde 37:953–955, 1981

Surmont DWA, Colardyn F, De Reuck J: Fatal complications of neuroleptic drugs: a clinico-pathological study of three cases. Acta Neurol Belg 84:75–83, 1984

Susman VL, Addonizio G: Reinduction of neuroleptic malignant syndrome by lithium. J Clin Psychopharmacol 7:339–341, 1987

Susman VL, Addonizio G: Recurrence of neuroleptic malignant syndrome. J Nerv Ment Dis 176:234–241, 1988

Swanson LW: An autoradiographic study of the efferent connections of the preoptic region of the rat. J Comp Neurol 167:227–256, 1976

Tacke U, Venalainen E: Heat stress and neuroleptic drugs. J Neurol Neurosurg Psychiatry 50:937–938, 1987

Takagi A: Chlorpromazine and skeletal muscle: a study of skinned single fibers of the guinea pig. Exp Neurol 73:477–486, 1981

Takagi A, Araki M: Release of calcium ion from sarcoplasmic reticulum (SR) of Duchenne muscular dystrophy (DMD) and malignant hyperthermia. Muscle Nerv 9:212, 1986

Tanner CM, Goetz CC, Klawans HL: Autonomic nervous system disorders, in Handbook of Parkinson's Disease. Edited by Koller WC. New York, Marcel Dekker, 1987, pp 145–170

Tarsy D: Neuroleptic-induced extrapyramidal reactions: classification, description, and diagnosis. Clin Neuropharmacol 6(Suppl 1):59–526, 1983

Taylor NE, Schwartz HI: Neuroleptic malignant syndrome following amoxipine overdose. J Nerv Ment Dis 176:249–251, 1988

Tenenbein M: The neuroleptic malignant syndrome: occurrence in a 15-year-old boy and recovery with bromocriptine therapy. Pediatric Neuroscience 12:161–164, 1986

Tesio I, Porta GL, Messa E: Cerebellar syndrome in lithium poisoning: a case of partial recovery. J Neurol Neurosurg Psychiatry 50:235, 1987

Thase ME, Shostak M: Rhabdomyolysis complicating rapid intramuscular neuroleptization. J Clin Psychopharmacol 4:46–48, 1984

Thomas CJ: Brain damage with lithium/haloperidol. Br J Psychiatry 134:552, 1979

Thomas C, Tatham A, Jakubowski S: Lithium/haloperidol combinations and brain damage. Lancet 1:626, 1982

Thompson TN: Malignant hyperthermia from phencyclidine. J Clin Psychiatry 40:327, 1979

Thorhton WE, Pray BJ: Lithium intoxication: a report of two cases. Can Psychiatr Assoc J 20:281–282, 1975

Tollefson G: A case of neuroleptic malignant syndrome: in-vitro muscle comparison with malignant hyperthermia. J Clin Psychopharmacol 1:266–270, 1982

Tollefson GD, Garvey MJ: The neuroleptic syndrome and central dopamine metabolites. J Clin Psychopharmacol 4:150–153, 1984

Tolsma FJ: Acute "pernicious" psychoses. Folia Psychiatrica Neurologica et Neurochirurgica Neerlandica 69:10–32, 1956

Tolsma FJ: The syndrome of acute pernicious psychosis. Psychiatr Neurol Neurochir 70:1–21, 1967

Tomson CRV: Neuroleptic malignant syndrome associated with inappropriate antidiuresis and psychogenic polydipsia. Br Med J 292:171, 1986

Tong TG, Benowitz NL, Becker CE, et al: Phencyclidine poisoning. JAMA 234:512–513, 1975

Toru M, Matsuda O, Makiguchi K, et al: Neuroleptic malignant syndrome-like state following a withdrawal of antiparkinsonian drugs. J Nerv Ment Dis 169:324–327, 1981

Towell A, Willner P, Muscat R: Dopamine autoreceptors in the ventral tegmental area show subsensitivity following withdrawal from chronic antidepressant drug treatment. Psychopharmacology 90:64–71, 1986

Tung H, Swainey FG: Severe neurotoxicity and lithium therapy. Clin Toxicol 13:479–486, 1986

Tupin JP, Schuller AB. Lithium and haloperidol incompatibility reviewed. Psychiatr J Univ Ottawa 3:245–251, 1978

Turski L, Havemann U, Kuschinsky K: The role of the substantia nigra in motility of the rat: muscular rigidity, body asymmetry and catalepsy after injection of morphine into the nigra. Neuropharmacology 22:1039–1048, 1983

Tyrer P, Alexander MS, Regan A: An extrapyramidal syndrome after lithium therapy. Br J Psychiatry 136:191–194, 1980

Ulus IH, Kiran BK, Ozkurt S: Involvement of central dopamine in the hyperthermia in rats produced by d-amphetamine. Pharmacology 13:309–316, 1975

Unger J, Decaux G, L'Hermite M: Rhabdomyolysis, acute renal failure, endocrine alterations and neurological sequelae in a case of lithium self poisoning. Acta Clin Belg 37:216–223, 1982

Ungvari GA: Treatment of neuroleptic malignant syndrome with dopamine hydrochloride: a case report. Pharmacopsychiatry 20:120–121, 1987

Utili R, Boitnott JK, Zimmerman HJ: Dantrolene-associated hepatic injury: incidence and character. Gastroenterology 72:610–616, 1977

Van Putten T: Why do schizophrenic patients refuse to take their drugs? Arch Gen Psychiatry 31:67–72, 1974

Varia IM, Taska RJ: The neuroleptic malignant syndrome: management and safety considerations. Medical Times 112:53–57, 1984

Venkatachari SAT, Pagala M, Herzlich B, et al: Effect of cocaine on neuromuscular function in isolated phrenic nerve diaphragm of mouse. FASEB J 2:A1138, 1988

Vergara J, Tsien RY, Delay M: Inositol 1, 4, 5-triphosphate: a possible chemical link in excitation-contraction coupling in muscle. Proc Natl Acad Sci USA 82:6352–6356, 1985

Verhoeven WMA, Elderson A, Westenberg HGM: Neuroleptic malignant syndrome: successful treatment with bromocriptine. Biol Psychiatry 20:680–684, 1985

Verilli MR, Salanga VD, Kozachuk WE, et al: Phenelzine toxicity responsive to dantrolene. Neurology 37:865–867, 1987

Vetulani J, Lebrecht U, Pilc A: Enhancement of responsiveness of the central serotonergic system and serotonin-2 receptor density in rat frontal cortex by electroconvulsive treatment. Eur J Pharmacol 76:81–85, 1981

Vincent FM, Zimmerman JE, Van Haren J: Neuroleptic malignant syndrome complicating closed head injury. Neurosurgery 18:190–193, 1986

Vizi ES, Illes P, Ronai A, et al: The effect of lithium on acetylcholine release and synthesis. Neuropharmacology 11:521–530, 1972

Voigt MM, Uhl GR: Neurotransmitter receptor alterations, in Handbook of Parkinson's Disease. Edited by Koller WC. New York, Marcel Dekker, 1987, pp 253–266

von Knorring L, Smigan L, Perris C, et al: Lithium and neuroleptic drugs in combination-effect on lithium RBC/plasma ratio. International Pharmacopsychiatry 17:287–292, 1982

von Muhlendahl KE, Krienke EG: Fenfluramine poisoning. Clin Toxicol 14:97–106, 1979

Wachtel TJ, Steele GH, Day JA: Natural history of fever following seizure. Arch Intern Med 147:1153–1155, 1987

Walenga RW, Opas EE, Feinstein MB: Differential effects of calmodulin antagonists on phospholipase A2 and C in thrombin-stimulated platelets. J Biol Chem 256:12523–12528, 1981

Wambebe C, Osuide G: Influence of some dopamine receptor agonists on pentobarbitone sleep in young chicks, in Advances in the Biosciences, Vol 37: Advances in Dopamine Research. Edited by Kohsaka M, Shohmori T, Tsukada Y, et al. Oxford, Pergamon, 1982, pp 363–368

Wand P, Kuschinsky K, Sontag KH: Morphine-induced muscular rigidity in rats. Eur J Pharmacol 24:189–193, 1973

Wandless I, Grimley-Evans J, Jackson M: Fever associated with metoclopramide-induced dystonia. Lancet 1:1255–1256, 1980

Ward A, Chaffman MO, Sorkin EM: Dantrolene: a review of its pharmacodynamic and pharmacokinetic properties, and therapeutic care of malignant hyperthermia, the neuroleptic malignant syndrome and an update of its use in muscle spasticity. Drugs 32:130–168, 1986

Wedzicha JA, Hoffbrand BI: Neuroleptic malignant syndrome and hyponatraemia. Lancet 2:963, 1984

Weiden P, Harrigan M: A clinical guide for diagnosing and managing patients with drug-induced dysphagia. Hosp Community Psychiatry 37:396–398, 1986

Weinberg S, Twersky RS: Neuroleptic malignant syndrome. Anesth Analg 62:848–850, 1983

Weinberger DR: Implications of normal brain development for the pathogenesis of schizophrenia. Arch Gen Psychiatry 44:660–669, 1987

Weinberger DR, Kelly MJ: Catatonia and malignant syndrome: a possible complication of neuroleptic administration. J Nerv Ment Dis 165:263–268, 1977

Weis J: On the hyperthermic response to d-amphetamine in the decapitated rat. Life Sci 13:475–484, 1973

Weiss B, Prozialeck WC, Wallace TL: Interaction of drugs with calmodulin: biochemical, pharmacological and clinical implications. Biochem Pharmacol 31:2217–2226, 1982

West AP, Meltzer HY: Paradoxical lithium neurotoxicity: a report of five cases and a hypothesis about risk for neurotoxicity. Am J Psychiatry 136:963–966, 1979

Wetli CV, Fishbain DA: Cocaine-induced psychosis and sudden death in recreational cocaine users. J Forensic Sci 30:873–880, 1985

Wheeler AH, Ziegler MG, Insel PA, et al: Episodic catatonia, hypertension, and tachycardia: elevated plasma catecholamines. Neurology 35:1053–1055, 1985

White K, Simpson G: Combined MAOI-tricyclic antidepressant treatment: a reevaluation. J Clin Psychopharmacol 1:264–282, 1981

White K, Simpson G: The combined use of MAOIs and tricyclics. J Clin Psychiatry 45(7, sec 2):67–69, 1984

White K, Pistole T, Boyd JL: Combined monoamine oxidase inhibitor-tricyclic antidepressant treatment: a pilot study. Am J Psychiatry 137:1422–1425, 1980

White PD: Treatment of neuroleptic malignant syndrome. Br J Psychiatry 144:437, 1984

Williams CH: Some observations on the etiology of the fulminant hyperthermia-stress syndrome. Perspect Biol Med 20:120–130, 1976

Williams M: Psychophysiologic responsiveness to psychologic stress in early chronic schizophrenia. Psychosom Med 15:456–462, 1953

Willner P: Dopamine and depression: a review of recent evidence, III: the effects of antidepressant treatments. Brain Research Review 6:237–246, 1983

Wilson LG: Viral encephalopathy mimicking functional psychosis. Am J Psychiatry 133:165–170, 1976

Wingard DW, Gatz EE: Some observations on stress-susceptible patients, in Second International Symposium on Malignant Hyperthermia. Edited by Aldrete JA, Britt BA. New York, Grune & Stratton, 1978, pp 363–372

Wirtshafter D, Asin KE, Kent EW: Nucleus accumbens lesions reduce amphetamine hyperthermia but not hyperactivity. Eur J Pharmacol 51:449–452, 1978

Wise TN: Heatstroke in three chronic schizophrenics: case reports and clinical considerations. Compr Psychiatry 14:263–267, 1973

Wooten GF: Neurochemistry, in Handbook of Parkinson's Disease. Edited by Koller WC. New York, Marcel Dekker, 1987, pp 237–253

Yacoub OF, Morrow DH: Malignant hyperthermia and ECT. Am J Psychiatry 143:1027–1029, 1986

Yamawaki S: A consideration on the pathophysiology of syndrome malin: three cases of successful treatment with dantrolene. Japanese Journal of Psychiatric Treatment 1:413–422, 1986

Yamawaki S, Lai H, Horita A: Dopaminergic and serotonergic mechanisms of thermoregulation: mediation of thermal effects of apomorphine and dopamine. J Pharmacol Exp Ther 227:383–388, 1983

Yassa R: A case of lithium-chlorpromazine interaction. J Clin Psychiatry 47:90–91, 1986

Yassa R, Archer J, Cordozo S: The long term effect of lithium carbonate on tardive dyskinesia. Can J Psychiatry 29:36–37, 1984

Yasukawa M, Hatakeyama Y, Yasukawa K, et al: A case of neuroleptic malignant syndrome with myoglobinuria. Masui 32:876–882, 1983

Yehuda S: The effects of d-amphetamine on dopaminergic regulated mechanisms of physiological and behavioral thermoregulation, in Current Developments in Psychopharmacology, Vol 5. Edited by Essman W, Vaczelci L. New York, SP Medical and Scientific Books, 1979, pp 125–171

Yehuda S, Frommer R: The possible role of dopamine in phenothiazine-induced hypothermia in rats: an application to DA hypothesis of schizophrenia. Int J Neurosci 7:67–72, 1977

Yehuda S, Wurtman RJ: Dopaminergic neurons in the nigro-striatal and mesolimbic pathways: mediation of specific effects of d-amphetamine. Eur J Pharmacol 30:154–158, 1975

Yoneda S, Tomioka H, Fukuyama M: Peripheral origin of plasma dopamine. Jpn Circ J 49:1028–1034, 1985

Young JPR, Lader MH, Hughes WC: Controlled trial of trimipramine, monoamine oxidase inhibitors, and combined treatment in depressed outpatients. Br Med J 2:1315–1317, 1979

Zalis EG, Pauley LF: Fatal amphetamine poisoning. Ann Intern Med 112:822–826, 1963

Zalis EG, Kaplan G, Lundberg GD, et al: Acute lethality of the amphetamines in dogs and its antagonism by curare. Proc Soc Exp Biol Med 118:557–561, 1965

Zalis EG, Lundberg GD, Knutson RA: The pathophysiology of acute amphetamine poisoning with pathologic considerations. J Pharm Exp Ther 158:115–127, 1967

Zamora-Quezada JC, Dinerman H, Stadecker MJ, et al: Muscle and skin infarction after free-basing cocaine (crack). Ann Intern Med 108:564–566, 1988

Zelman S, Guillan R: Heatstroke in phenothiazine-treated patients: a report of three fatalities. Am J Psychiatry 126:1787–1790, 1970

Zetin M, Plon L, DeAntonio M: MAOI reaction with powdered protein dietary supplement. J Clin Psychiatry 48:499, 1987

Zubenko G, Pope HG Jr: Management of a case of neuroleptic malignant syndrome with bromocriptine. Am J Psychiatry 140:1619–1620, 1983